Near Misses in Pediatric Anesthesia

John G. Brock-Utne

Near Misses in Pediatric Anesthesia

Second Edition

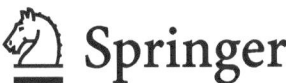 Springer

John G. Brock-Utne, MD, PhD, FFA(SA)
Department of Anesthesia
Stanford University
Stanford, CA, USA

ISBN 978-1-4614-7039-7   ISBN 978-1-4614-7040-3 (eBook)
DOI 10.1007/978-1-4614-7040-3
Springer New York Heidelberg Dordrecht London

Library of Congress Control Number: 2013935495

Printed on acid-free paper

Springer is part of Springer Science+Business Media (www.springer.com)

Foreword

After 40 years of working as an anesthesiologist, I occasionally fool myself into believing I have "seen it all." The truth: no one ever sees every possible clinical scenario. Unique presentations can occur whether it's your first day of anesthesia residency training or the last day of a long and eventful career. Only by sharing experiences can everyone learn from them. Dr. John Brock-Utne has had his share of unique cases. However, unlike most of us, he has recorded and collected them in this very useful book. Combining his talents as both a superb clinician and an award-winning teacher, he is able to describe a clinical situation, explain his thoughts in arriving at a diagnosis, and then describe how to apply the appropriate management. Thus, even after 40 years of practicing anesthesiology, I still continue to learn from him. Just as he has been a source of knowledge and information for me and the faculty and house staff at Stanford University, the reader can also now benefit from his knowledgeable and entertaining approach to the anesthetic management of unusual cases.

Stanford, CA, USA   Jay B. Brodsky

Preface to the Second Edition

Dear Reader,

Some of you may have read the first edition of *Near Misses in Pediatric Anesthesia*, published by Heinemann-Butterworth in 1999. I thought this would be the only edition. But thanks to Shelley Reinhardt, Senior Editor, Springer Science+Business Media, the first edition has been revived. This is therefore the second edition with 40 new additional cases. The original 47 cases have been revised and updated. I hope you will find the cases interesting and educational.

Again, each individual case starts with a short introduction. You are provided with the essential information to solve the problem. On the following page, you are given the solution and suggested management.

As with the first edition, the management of the cases may be controversial. Hence, I hope they will provide a basis for a discussion between a faculty member and an anesthesia resident, an anesthesia assistant, a CRNA, or a medical student as to other and possibly better alternative solutions.

Anesthesia has become much safer since I started my training in Oslo, Norway, on July 1, 1970. Now, 43 years later, I often cover up the anesthesia monitor, including information from the anesthesia machine about tidal volume, etc., when I work with new trainees. I say, "Now give the anesthetic. This is what it was like when I started." The response is utter disbelief. But the reason I do this is to stress the importance of examining your patients. This is especially true when the patient's vital signs are unstable. Remember not to solely rely on the monitors, as they are only an aid in your ongoing clinical assessment of your patient's well-being.

To paraphrase Hippocrates:

The art is long,
Life is short,
Experiments perilous,
Decisions difficult.

Stanford, CA, USA   John G. Brock-Utne

Preface to the First Edition

Anesthesiologists sometimes face difficult decisions in "near miss" situations. The risk-to-benefit ratios in these cases are often unknown. Fortunately, near misses occur rarely. The near misses reported in this book come mostly from my 30 years experience in clinical anesthesia in the United States, Scandinavia, and South Africa.

Each of the 47 cases starts with a short introduction to the clinical problem. The reader is provided with all the essential information necessary to prevent a disaster. The next page provides a solution and analysis of the problem, makes recommendations, and provides references for further reading.

Some of the sequences in the management of these cases may be controversial. As such, they may form the basis for a teaching discussion between a faculty member and a resident in anesthesiology. Most of all, the book is designed to alert the reader to various precarious situations that can arise and how best to prevent or deal with them. To paraphrase Hippocrates:

The art is long,
Life is short,
Experiments perilous,
Decisions difficult.

Stanford, CA, USA   John G. Brock-Utne

Acknowledgments

I would like to acknowledge my many colleagues around the world who have contributed to this book through our case reports and discussions regarding the many problematic cases:

Aitchison J, Andrews AD, Angelotti T, Barclay R, Bernstein O, Bland BAR, Bolton P, Bosenberg AT, Botz G, Brodsky JB, Brun C, Bushell E, Ceranski J, Chen K, Chu LF, Claure RE, Cochran M, Collins JS, DeBasttista C, Diachun CAB, Dimopoulos GE, Dow TGB, Downing JW, Eide AM, Eng MR, Fisher SP, Ganguly K, Giffard R, Habibi A, Haddow GR, Hammer G, Hester J, van der Heyden A, Hilton G, Hold AR, Holloway AM, Honkanen A, Humphrey D, Jaffe RA, Kim A, Krane EJ, Kingston HGG, Lemmens HJM, Lin YC, Lopes JR, Luckin P, Macario A, MacGillivray RG, Mallat AM, Mariano ER, Mark JB, Moll V, Moshal MG, Moynihan RJ, Naicker S, Naidu N, Naidu R, Odell JA, Pond D, Ratner E, Reid CS, Roberson J, Robins B, Robles B, Rubin J, Schmiesing CA, Sculte-Steinberg O, Silver L, Vogel T, Wang R, Welman S, Wu TT, and Zumaran AA.

I am also indebted to Dr. Jay B. Brodsky (Medical Director of the Stanford Operating Rooms) for kindly agreeing to write a foreword for this book; Dr. Richard A. Jaffe for his friendship and encouragement; Shelley Reinhardt, Joanna Perey, and Maureen Pierce (Springer) for all their help and support; and last, but not least, to my wife Sue, our three boys, their wives, and our five grandsons and one granddaughter.

John G. Brock-Utne

Contents

Chapter 1
Case 1: Upper Gastrointestinal Endoscopy Under General Anesthesia

A 23-month-old, previously healthy girl (16 kg) is scheduled for endoscopy and removal of an esophageal web. Her medical history is unremarkable except for mild dysphasia. Her vital signs are normal.

General anesthesia is induced via face mask using sevoflurane 1–4 % in nitrous oxide and 30 % oxygen after all necessary monitoring equipment is placed on the child. After the child is asleep, an intravenous (IV) line is inserted, and 0.15 mg atropine and 1.6 mg vecuronium are administered to facilitate tracheal intubation with a 5-mm internal diameter (i.d.) tracheal tube. Breath sounds are equal bilaterally, and a leak around the tube in the trachea is present at 20 cm H_2O peak inflation pressure. The endotracheal tube (ETT) is securely taped. The patient's lungs are hand ventilated using peak inspiratory pressures of 15–35 cm H_2O. The patient is draped from the neck down, and the endoscopist places the gastroscope into the esophagus without difficulty. A few minutes later, the lungs become less compliant, and the child's blood pressure (BP) decreases over a 5-min period from 90/50 to 70/35 mmHg. The electrocardiogram (ECG) is judged to be normal, and the heart rate increases from 110 to 130 beats per minute [1] (bpm) with a regular sinus rhythm. The capnograph demonstrates a CO_2 waveform. The shape has not changed; however, the peak airway pressure now increases from 22 to 38 cm H_2O. The peripheral oxygen saturation decreases from 100 % to 86 %. You do the following:

1. Increase the FIO_2 to 100 %.
2. Continue hand ventilation.
3. Ascertain the correct position of the ETT.
4. Pass a suction catheter successfully down the whole length of the ETT.

Question

No improvement is seen. What will you do, and what is the cause of the dilemma?

J.G. Brock-Utne, *Near Misses in Pediatric Anesthesia*,
DOI 10.1007/978-1-4614-7040-3_1, © Springer Science+Business Media New York 2013

Solution

The patient was undraped so her chest could be examined. The epigastrium was seen to be markedly distended. Unknown to the anesthesiologist, the endoscopist had injected air to dilate the esophagus and the stomach for better visualization. With gastric decompression, the patient's respiratory and cardiovascular parameters immediately returned to normal. The case proceeded without difficulty, and the patient made an uneventful recovery.

Discussion

This problem has been noted in both pediatric [1] and adult cases [2]. In the adult case, severe respiratory distress occurred during upper gastrointestinal endoscopy in a 30-year-old man. The procedure was performed under local anesthesia and sedation, and the cause of the respiratory distress was thought to be excess air insufflation into a stomach positioned within the chest through a hiatal hernia. The case reported here differs in that the patient was anesthetized with a normally positioned stomach. Excess insufflation of air into the esophagus dilated the stomach and markedly decreased chest compliance. The desaturation noted in this case most likely reflected the effect of ventilation/perfusion (V/Q) mismatch in a lung being compressed by a distended stomach.

Excessive gastric air insufflation has also been reported in neonates with tracheoesophageal fistulas, at times associated with cardiac arrest presumed secondary to the same mechanism [3]. Hence, use of a preoperative gastrostomy tube has been recommended in these cases to vent excess air.

This case would not have occurred had the anesthesiologist had the opportunity to observe the child's abdomen. It is not essential to cover patients for nonsterile procedures.

Recommendation

The epigastrium must be seen at all times during upper gastrointestinal endoscopy to prevent the possibility of excessive gastric distension.

References

1. Brock-Utne JG, Moynihan RJ. Patient draping contributing to the near disaster (desaturation during endoscopy in a 2-year-old) (case report). Paediatr Anaesth. 1992;2:333–4.
2. Narendranathan M, Kalam A. Respiratory distress during endoscopy—report of an unusual case. Postgrad Med J. 1987;6:805–6.
3. Baraka A, Slim M. Cardiac arrest during IPPV in a newborn with tracheoesophageal fistula. Anesthesiology. 1970;32:564–5.

Chapter 2
Case 2: Sudden Anesthesia System Failure

A 1-year-old patient, American Society of Anesthesiologists (ASA) physical status II, is to undergo removal of a cerebral tumor under general anesthesia. An anesthesia machine and breathing system check is performed before the patient's arrival. Noninvasive monitors are placed, and after preoxygenation the patient is anesthetized in a routine manner. Invasive monitors are placed, the operating table is turned 180°, and the operation begins. About 2 h into the operation, the surgeon requests that the operating table be elevated. Three to five minutes later, warning lights flash on the anesthesia machine (Narkomed 2 B, North American Drager). The warning indicates low minute volume, apnea, and no ventilation of the patient. The rotameters show adequate flow of oxygen and nitrous oxide, and the oxygen pipeline pressure is 50 psi.

Manual ventilation is attempted using the anesthesia machine's collapsible breathing bag but is unsuccessful because no air fills the bag despite using the oxygen flush control button. You do the following:

1. Provide self-inflatable bag ventilation. Confirm bilateral air entry. Keep the patient's oxygen saturation and vital signs stable.
2. Call for assistance.
3. Search for a cause of the breathing system failure in the anesthesia machine.

Question

You and your colleagues find nothing wrong with the machine. So what could be the cause of this dilemma?

J.G. Brock-Utne, *Near Misses in Pediatric Anesthesia*,
DOI 10.1007/978-1-4614-7040-3_2, © Springer Science+Business Media New York 2013

Solution

The cause of the acute distress was a kinked and compressed fresh gas flow tube between the railing of the operating room table and the bottom of the inspiratory pipe on the absorber (Fig. 2.1). This occurred when the operating table was raised [1].

Recommendation

The fresh gas flow tube from the anesthesia machine to absorber should always be short and not hanging loose. It should always be positioned behind the upright support brace (D) of the absorber, thereby preventing a kink in the tube.

A self-inflatable bag should be available in every operating room.

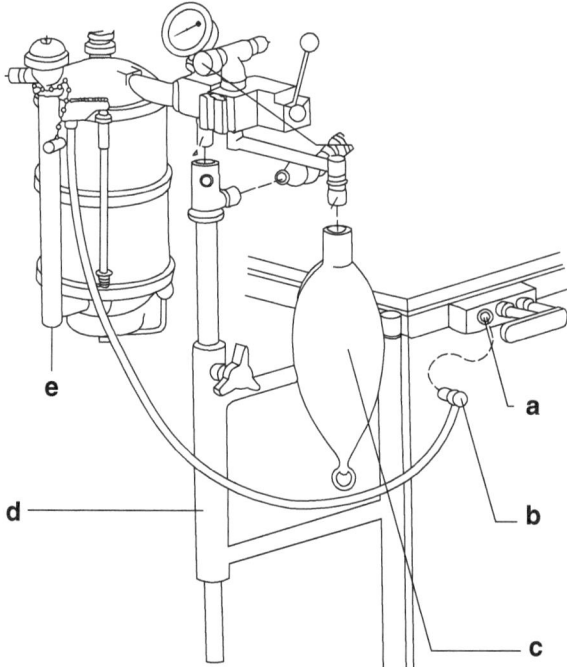

Fig. 2.1 (**a**) Fresh gas-locking device. (**b**) Fresh gas hose with 15-mm fitting. (**c**) Breathing bag. (**d**) Upright support brace. (**e**) Inspiratory pipe of the absorber

Reference

1. Silver L, Lopes N, Brock-Utne JG. Raising the operating table causing a sudden anesthesia system obstruction. Anesth Analg. 1996;82:1107–8.

Chapter 3
Case 3: Broviac Catheter Placement in a Neonatal Intensive Care Unit

A 43-day-old (1.3-kg) girl born at 27 weeks is scheduled for a Broviac catheter replacement in the neonatal intensive care unit (NICU). She is in the NICU because of respiratory failure, bronchopulmonary dysplasia, right lower lobe pneumonia, and sepsis. She has failed extubation twice in the past due to postextubation stridor and desaturation. The day before surgery, the patient was intubated with a 2.5 endotracheal tube (ETT) by the NICU staff and ventilated for 12 h before surgery. A large leak has been suspected around the endotracheal tube (ETT), as the nurse has noted hearing the patient cough and cry. At present, the ventilator is working and the settings include an FIO_2 of 30 %, respiratory rate of 14, and the pressure setting of 24/5. The patient's vital signs include a respiratory rate of 60, heart rate of 150 bpm, and oxygen saturation by pulse oximetry of 92–95 %. Her gastric tube is in place and open to air. Coarse breath sounds are heard bilaterally without evidence of leakage around the ETT. Standard monitoring devices are placed except for an end-tidal CO_2 monitor, which is not available. A preoperative radiography of the chest had been taken earlier in the morning but is unavailable for viewing.

Immediately after induction of anesthesia with intravenous (IV) pancuronium and fentanyl, the patient's oxygen saturation falls precipitously to 0, with a decrease in heart rate to the 1990s and with ST segment elevations. The patient is immediately ventilated via the ETT with 100 % oxygen. The breath sounds remain coarse and unchanged. A new pulse oximetry probe is placed by a nurse to rule out probe malfunction. There is no improvement in the oxygen saturation reading. No abdominal distension is noticed. IV atropine is administered to treat the bradycardia, and a call for help is made. Noninvasive blood pressure (BP) measurements remain within normal limits throughout this time. The heart rate responds to atropine, and the ST segment elevation partially resolves over the next minute.

Question

Oxygen saturation is still inadequate. What will you do now?

J.G. Brock-Utne, *Near Misses in Pediatric Anesthesia*,
DOI 10.1007/978-1-4614-7040-3_3, © Springer Science+Business Media New York 2013

Solutions

1. Perform a direct laryngoscopy to confirm correct placement of the ETT. In this case, the ETT is found to be in the esophagus. The ETT is placed in the trachea and the lungs ventilated with a rapid rise in oxygen saturation.
2. If the ETT was found to be in the trachea, transillumination of the chest with a torch could eliminate a possible pneumothorax.

Discussion

The preoperative detection of the esophageal-placed ETT proved elusive in this case [1]. Physical examination was not helpful in detecting esophageal intubation because the patient's breath sounds were transmitted throughout the thorax and abdomen. Even if we had reviewed the chest radiography preoperatively, we probably would have missed the esophageal positioning of the ETT because attention would have been focused primarily on the relative position of the tip of the ETT and the carina. Because the patient appeared to be adequately ventilated and oxygenated before induction of anesthesia, a pre-existing esophageal position ETT was not an obvious cause of postinduction desaturation.

Recommendation

Clamping or kinking the nasogastric tube while the patient was being ventilated with the intensive care unit (ICU) ventilator could have led to gastric distension within a few minutes. In our case, this was not done. We believe that the gastric distension was not seen because the patient's stomach was continuously decompressed by the nasogastric tube. The nasogastric tube therefore prevented a buildup of gastric pressure that could have led to an obvious degree of abdominal distension and the sounding of the high pressure alarm on the ventilator.

Reference

1. Crockett DE, Tays R, Brock-Utne JG. Twelve hours of gastric ventilation. A recipe for disaster (a suggested remedy). Paediatr Anaesth. 1998;8:171–3.

Suggested Reading

Anderson K, Schultz-Labahn T. Oesophageal intubation can be undetected by auscultation of the chest. Acta Anaesthesiol Scand. 1994;38:580–2.

Bhende MS, Thompson AE, Cook DR, Saville AL. Validity of a disposable end-tidal CO_2 detector in verifying ETT placement in infants and children. Ann Emerg Med. 1992;21:142–5.

Bhende MS, Thompson AE, Orr RA. Utility of an end-tidal carbon dioxide detector during stabilization and transport of critically ill children. Pediatrics. 1992;89:1042–4.

Holland R, Webb RK, Runciman WB. The Australian incident monitoring study. System failure: an analysis of 2000 incident reports. Anaesth Intensive Care. 1993;21:684–95.

Unseld H. Unrecognized esophageal intubation. Consideration of prevention in a case. Anaesthesist. 1988;37:198–201.

Chapter 4
Case 4: Occluded Reinforced (Armored) Endotracheal Tube

An 8-year-old boy is presented for a major ear, nose, and throat (ENT) procedure. A reinforced endotracheal tube (ETT) (Mallinckrodt, St. Louis, MO) is used to secure the airway after induction of general anesthesia. Normally, these tubes are removed at the end of the procedure once the tracheostomy has been performed. In this case, however, due to surgical reasons, a tracheostomy is not done, and the patient is taken to the intensive care unit (ICU) with the reinforced ETT in place. You decide to leave the ETT in the trachea and to ventilate the child mechanically overnight because he exhibits marked head and neck edema after 10 h of surgery. The possibility of potential severe laryngeal edema makes you decide not to change the reinforced ETT with a standard ETT over a tube changer. The next morning, on awakening from the sedation, the patient bites down vigorously on the reinforced ETT. Due to the nature of the reinforced ETT, the lumen becomes completely occluded and will not re-expand. The patient cannot breathe nor can the lungs be ventilated. This results in oxygen desaturation to 80 %. Cyanosis becomes evident. The jaw can easily be opened.

Question

What will you do now?

J.G. Brock-Utne, *Near Misses in Pediatric Anesthesia*,
DOI 10.1007/978-1-4614-7040-3_4, © Springer Science+Business Media New York 2013

Solution

The best solution is to use a hemostat to manipulate the reinforced ETT into its original shape by placing the hemostat at 90° to the occlusion. In this way, you open the ETT lumen [1].

You could also cut the ETT below the obstruction and pass a tube changer or a gum-elastic bougie through the cut ETT. When that is done, you could pass a new non-reinforceable ETT into the trachea [2].

Recommendation

A hard bit block, not an oral airway, should always be used with an armored ETT [1–3]. This is to prevent the occlusion of the ETT and even biting the ETT in half [4].

References

1. Vogel T, Brock-Utne JG. Solution to an occluded reinforced (armored) endotracheal tube. Am J Anesthesiol. 1997;2:58–61.
2. Robles B, Hester J, Brock-Utne JG. Remember the gum-elastic bougie at extubation. J Clin Anesth. 1993;5:329–31.
3. King H-K, Lewis K. Guedel oropharyngeal airway does not prevent patient biting on the endotracheal tube. Anaesth Intensive Care. 1996;24:6.
4. Kong CS. A small child can bite through an armored tracheal tube. Anaesthesia. 1995;50:263.

Suggested Reading

Adamson DH. A problem of prolonged oral intubation: case report. Can J Anaesth. 1971;18:213–4.
Dempsey GA, Barrett PJ. Hazard with the reinforced laryngeal mask airway. Anaesthesia. 1995;50:660–1.
Gemma M, Ferrazza C. "Dental trauma" to oral airways. Can J Anaesth. 1989;36:951.
Hoffman CO, Swanson GA. Oral reinforced endotracheal tube crushed and perforated from biting. Anesth Analg. 1989;69:548–53.
Hull JM. Occlusion of armoured tubes. Anesthesia. 1989;44:790.
Martens P. Persistent narrowing of an armoured tube. Anaesthesia. 1992;47:716–7.
McTaggart RA, Shustack A, Noseworthy T, Johnston R. Another cause of obstruction in an armored endotracheal tube. Anesthesiology. 1983;59:164.
Peck MJ, Neddleman SM. Reinforced endotracheal tube obstruction. Anesth Analg. 1994;79:193.
Singh B, Srivastava SK, Chhabra B. Reinforced orotracheal tube obstruction: pharyngeal or oral? Anesth Analg. 1994;79:193–4.
Spiess BD, Rothenberg DM, Buckley S. Complete airway obstruction of armored endotracheal tubes. Anesth Analg. 1991;73:95–6.

Chapter 5
Case 5: The Too-Small Rigid Bronchoscope

A 12-year-old boy (70 kg) with right bronchial obstruction is scheduled for fiber-optic bronchoscopy and rigid bronchoscopy with laser treatment. His history and physical examination are unremarkable. A tumor of unknown origin is thought to partially obstruct the right main bronchus. The patient has no known drug or food allergies and no previous anesthesia/surgery. The family history is negative for anesthesia-related complications. The patient is classified as American Society of Anesthesiologists physical status II (ASA 2).

The patient is brought to the operating room. The vital signs include blood pressure (BP) of 100/60, regular heart rate of 80 bpm, and 100 % oxygen saturation by pulse oximetry. After an intravenous (IV) line is placed, the patient is given propofol and vecuronium in usual doses. The trachea is intubated with a No. 7 endotracheal tube (ETT), and the fiber-optic bronchoscopy is performed without any complications. Thereafter, the ETT is removed and a rigid bronchoscope (size 3.5 mm i.d. [internal diameter], 5 mm outer diameter [o.d.], 5.7 mm; Karl Storz, Germany) is inserted. This scope is obviously too small for the trachea, but the appropriate size is unavailable. A large leak is created. It becomes impossible to oxygenate the patient adequately. You inform the surgeon and suggest that the procedure be aborted and attempted again in the future when the appropriate equipment is available. This suggestion is declined by the surgeon who suggests jet ventilation. Unfortunately, the latter is not available. The surgeon still wants to proceed.

Question

What will you do to perform this anesthetic safely?

J.G. Brock-Utne, *Near Misses in Pediatric Anesthesia*,   13
DOI 10.1007/978-1-4614-7040-3_5, © Springer Science+Business Media New York 2013

Solution

The problem can easily rectified by packing the pharynx with a 2-in. moist vaginal pack [1]. I have used this several times with success.

Discussion

In these cases, the availability of a vaginal pack can be life saving. These packs are also useful in cases in which an endotracheal cuff develops a leak after a successful but very difficult intubation. The reluctance to remove a correctly placed ETT in these circumstances is understandable. Even changing the ETT over a tube changer may be considered potentially dangerous. Packing the throat in these cases may prove the better part of valor. The pack will "buy time" to stabilize the patient's vital signs. I have used this technique in the emergency room many times.

Recommendation

The throat packs come in two sizes: 1 or 2 in. Moisten the pack in water and squeeze the water out. Tie a single knot in what will be the distal end of the pack. Having done this, you know the pack is fully removed when you take the pack out.

Since packs are often not placed into the throat, it is imperative to remember its presence at the time of extubation. As a reminder, write "PACK" on two pieces of tape and place them on the patient's forehead and on the ETT.

Reference

1. Vickery IM, Burton GW. Throat packs for surgery. Anaesthesia. 1997;32:565–72.

Chapter 6
Case 6: Anaphylaxis, Anaphylactoid Reaction, or What Was It?

A 14-year-old healthy girl (weight 60 kg, height 150 cm) with idiopathic scoliosis is scheduled for a spinal instrumentation with Harrington rod placement for cosmetic reasons. She has no known drug or food allergies. The patient and her family have no history of anesthesia-related complications. The patient is taking no medications, is classified as American Society of Anesthesiologists physical status I (ASA 1), and has a hematocrit of 36 %. (She has donated 1 unit of blood.) In the operating room, the following drugs are given intravenously: midazolam (1 mg), thiopental (250 mg), fentanyl (100 μ[mu]g), and vecuronium (6 mg). An erythematous rash confined to the upper body is noted within 2 min of induction. Vital signs do not change. Her trachea is intubated without difficulty. Anesthesia is maintained with nitrous oxide 70 % in oxygen and isoflurane 0.6–0.8 %. The patient is given cefazolin (1 g) without any adverse effect over a 10-min period after being given a 100-mg test dose. Invasive monitors are placed. Fifteen minutes after induction, the rash has completely resolved. Three hundred milliliters of her own blood is collected from the central line before surgery for autotransfusion. The patient is turned prone and surgery commences. Ninety minutes after induction of anesthesia, the surgeon complains that the patient is moving. At this time, the vital signs are mean arterial pressure (MAP): 70 mmHg; heart rate: 72; and central venous pressure (CVP): 8 mmHg. The total IV crystalloids given at that time is 1,000 ml and the estimated surgical blood loss is 500 ml. Immediately after the second dose of vecuronium (2 mg), the patient becomes severely hypotensive with an MAP of 25, a pulse of 140 bpm, and an oxygen saturation of 86 %. There is no change in peak inspiratory pressure. No expiratory stridor or wheezing is heard. There is a decrease in the end-tidal CO_2 from 30 to 18 mmHg. No rash is noted on face or arms. The rest of the body is draped and is unavailable for examination.

Question

What will you do?

J.G. Brock-Utne, *Near Misses in Pediatric Anesthesia*, 15
DOI 10.1007/978-1-4614-7040-3_6, © Springer Science+Business Media New York 2013

Solution

Call a code, increase FIO_2 to 100 %, hand ventilate, and give vasoactive agents. In this case, 15 mg of ephedrine (the only pressor already drawn up) was given, and the MAP rose to 88 mmHg within 45 s and slowly returned to pre-event levels (Fig. 6.1). An arterial blood gas taken 5 min after the ephedrine showed a pH of 7.38, PCO_2 of 36 mmHg, and PO_2 of 143 mmHg (FIO_2 of 50 %). The surgery continued and an intraoperative wake-up test was done successfully. Further neuromuscular relaxation was achieved with pancuronium without any adverse effects. The operation proceeded uneventfully and the endotracheal tube (ETT) was removed at the end of surgery with the patient awake, cooperative, and breathing spontaneously. No neurodeficit or rash was seen.

Discussion

The sudden hypotension was most likely due to relative hypovolemia because of the patient's rapid response to ephedrine (15 mg). Forgetting to take into account the blood taken from the CVP line as part of the blood loss was a mistake. In fact, the blood loss was at least 800 ml. When the patient's muscles relaxed after the second dose of vecuronium, there was no compensatory mechanism.

Another cause could have been an air embolism, but no nitrogen was seen on the Rascal mass spectrometer.

The neuromuscular-blocking agents are a group of drugs known to stimulate histamine release. Cutaneous reactions are frequent, and anaphylactoid and anaphylactic reactions also occur but are uncommon. Vecuronium has been promoted as an agent that does not cause histamine release in clinical doses [1]. However, there has been one case report of anaphylactic shock including bronchospasms [2], one case of bronchospasm [3], and two cases of histamine release due to the drug [4, 5]. Fisher and Munroe [6] think that life-threatening anaphylactoid reactions to muscle relaxants occur more commonly than previously thought.

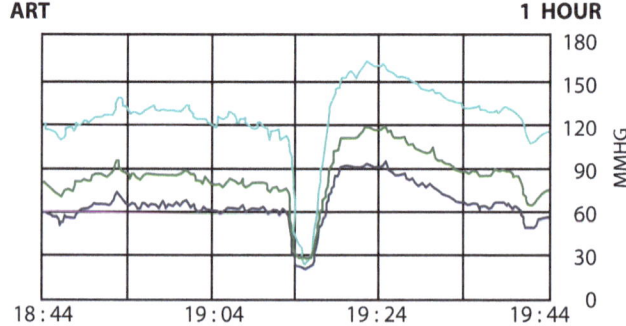

Fig. 6.1 Transient hypotension due to hypovolemia, corrected with 15 mg of ephedrine

Recommendations

1. Blood from a CVP line for later transfusion should, at the time of withdrawal, be recorded as blood loss.
2. It is essential to analyze the reasons for any hypotension and not to jump to inappropriate conclusions. In this case the patient could have been labeled as allergic to vecuronium, for example.
3. If allergies from any cause are expected, it is imperative to have allergy testing performed postoperatively [7].

References

1. Bowman WC. A new non-depolarizing neuromuscular blocking drug. Trends Pharmacol Sci. 1980;1:263–6.
2. Conil C, Bornet JL, Jean-Noel M, Conil JM, Brouchet A. Choc anaphylactique au pancuronium et au vecuronium [Anaphylactoid reactions to pancuronium and vecuronium.]. Ann Fr Anesth Reanim. 1985;4:241–3.
3. O'Callaghan AC, Scadding G, Watkins J. Bronchospasm following the use of vecuronium. Anaesthesia. 1986;41:940–2.
4. Clayton DG, Watkins J. Histamine release with vecuronium. Anaesthesia. 1984;39:1143–4.
5. Lavery GG, Hewitt AJ, Kenny NT. Possible histamine release after vecuronium. Anaesthesia. 1985;40:389–90.
6. Fisher M, Munro I. Life-threatening anaphylactoid reactions to muscle relaxants. Anesth Analg. 1983;62:559–64.
7. Intradermal tests for allergy [editorial]. Anaesth Intensive Care. 1976;4:95.

Chapter 7
Case 7: Generalized Convulsions After Regional Anesthesia

A 16-year-old boy (50 kg) is admitted in the early hours of the morning for repair of a cut right ulnar nerve. He is under the influence of alcohol and states that he has neither eaten nor drunk anything for 5 h. His vital signs are stable and his hemoglobin is 11 g%. He has no fixed address and denies any medical problems or illicit drug use. He comes to the operating room with an intravenous (IV) infusion of lactated Ringer's solution. He has received a total of 1 l since admission 2 h earlier. At 4:00 a.m., a supraclavicular brachial plexus block is performed with a mixture of 1.5 mg/kg (20 ml) bupivacaine 0.5 % and 1.5 mg/kg lidocaine 1 % (10 ml). At 4:20 a.m., surgery starts. Five minutes later (4:25 a.m.), the patient develops what appear to be generalized convulsions. However, he is breathing, and oxygen saturation remains within acceptable limits above 95 %. His heart rate is 94 regular, and his blood pressure (BP) is 140/90.

You provide oxygen via face mask and wonder what to do next as the surgeons have stopped working because the patient, but not the injured arm, is moving.

Question

What is the possible diagnosis and what will you do?

Differential Diagnosis

1. Toxic reaction to the local anesthetic drugs. Unlikely. The length of time from the injection of the drugs to the onset of convulsions is too long even for a delayed onset caused by slow absorption (25 min).
2. Undiagnosed epileptic. Unlikely. He did not show the classic signs of an epileptic convulsion such as incontinence and tongue biting.
3. Hypoglycemic coma caused by excessive and prolonged alcohol intake. Likely.

Solution

You decide on the third option and inject 50 % dextrose solution with good effects. The patient stops convulsing and becomes rational.

Discussion

In a previous case, it was reported that a 22-year-old man with a history of excessive alcohol intake developed delayed convulsions after a regional block [1]. In that case, the convulsions subsided over a 10-min period after administration of IV glucose. The patient's blood glucose level after receiving 60 ml of 50 % dextrose was 2.5 mmol/l (normal fasting levels, 3.33–6.60 mmol/l). He made an uneventful recovery, and his ulnar nerve was repaired under the supraclavicular block.

Recommendations

1. Excessive alcohol intake can cause hypoglycemia. If this diagnosis is missed and the patient is given a general anesthetic without glucose or wrongly treated for a toxic reaction to local anesthetics (e.g., paralyzing and ventilating the patient), serious brain damage could ensue.
2. Chronic alcohol intoxication is not age restricted.

Reference

1. Naidu R, Brock-Utne JG. Generalized convulsion following regional anesthesia—a pertinent lesson. Anesth Analg. 1988;67:1192.

Suggested Reading

Wilson NM, Brown PM, Juul SM, Prestwich SA, Sönksen PH. Glucose turnover and metabolic and hormonal changes in ethanol-induced hypoglycaemia. BMJ. 1981;282:849–53.

Chapter 8
Case 8: Hypotension During Microdiscectomy

A 16-year-old girl (American Society of Anesthesiologists physical status I [ASA 1]) is scheduled for a bilateral L4–L5 microdiscectomy. Aside from her back complaint, she is healthy with no known allergies. She has donated 1 unit of her own blood. She weighs 67 kg and measures 5 ft 4 in.; her starting hematocrit (Hct) is 35 %. In the operating room, after standard monitoring is placed, she is anesthetized in a routine manner and turned prone for the surgery. Ninety minutes into the surgery, with blood loss estimated to be 200 ml, sudden onset of tachycardia from 76 beats per minute (bpm) to 120 bpm occurs. The blood pressure (BP) decreases from a mean arterial pressure (MAP) of 80 mmHg to 50 mmHg. The surgeon is informed. He sees no evidence of any acute blood loss. The hypotension is treated with ephedrine and 750 ml of albumin with good result. An intraoperative Hct taken after the event is 25 %. As a precaution, a 16-gauge intravenous (IV) line is placed in her external jugular vein, and her right radial artery is cannulated. One hour later, the surgeon finishes the operation. Estimated blood loss per suction bottle is 600 ml, and a repeat Hct is 21 %. The vital signs are stable. The surgeon wants a quick changeover, so he can start his next case.

1. You decide to delay the next case and keep the patient anesthetized in the supine position with an endotracheal tube (ETT) in situ. You are concerned about a potential catastrophic hypovolemic situation.
2. You give the autologous unit.
3. You measure the abdominal girth regularly.
4. One hour later, you terminate the general anesthesia and take the patient to the recovery room. She is observed there for 2 h.
5. The family is informed of the high probability of a severe bleed from an epidural vein.
6. With vital signs stable (Hct at 22 %), you discharge the patient to the ward. No abdominal distension is seen.
7. The patient is discharged home 3 days later with no back pain.

Two weeks later, the patient is airlifted back to the hospital by helicopter in hypovolemic shock. At operation, a traumatic iliac artery aneurysm is repaired.

J.G. Brock-Utne, *Near Misses in Pediatric Anesthesia*,
DOI 10.1007/978-1-4614-7040-3_8, © Springer Science+Business Media New York 2013

Question

What should you have done differently?

Solution

In this case, a computed tomography (CT) scan of the patient's abdomen should have been performed postoperatively to rule out a retroperitoneal bleed. The aneurysm could then have been repaired immediately.

Recommendation

The lesson from this case is that unexplained, severe, intraoperative hypotension should be taken seriously.[1]

---

[1] This case is similar to the case of Jeff Chandler, a famous actor from Los Angeles, who died from hypovolemic shock in the recovery room after a laminectomy. The cause of death was a surgically traumatized iliac artery.

Chapter 9
Case 9: Intraoperative Hypotension in a Patient Receiving Chronic Steroids

A 4-year-old boy (12 kg) presents for surgical excision of a kidney tumor. His history includes severe asthma that is treated with prednisone, 2 mg per day. Two days before surgery, he was given bronchodilator therapy to optimize pulmonary function. The patient is anesthetized by an inhalation induction with sevoflurane. An intravenous (IV) line is inserted, and vecuronium and hydrocortisone 50 mg are given. Endotracheal intubation is performed uneventfully. Anesthesia is maintained with fentanyl and isoflurane in an oxygen-air mixture. Surgical resection of the kidney proves difficult, and surgical bleeding ensues. Blood loss (1,000 ml) is replaced. The internal jugular vein and right radial lines are cannulated. Bleeding continues (blood loss now 1,500 ml). Blood and crystalloid are given. A moderate acidosis (base excess 7) and a low serum calcium are corrected. Eventually the bleeding is under control and the central venous pressure (CVP) is 10 mmHg, but the blood pressure (BP) decreases precipitously, despite multiple IV doses of ephedrine, phenylephrine, epinephrine, and dopamine infusion to support the BP.

Question

While you are considering a pulmonary artery catheter and giving magnesium, is there anything else you would do?

J.G. Brock-Utne, *Near Misses in Pediatric Anesthesia*,
DOI 10.1007/978-1-4614-7040-3_9, © Springer Science+Business Media New York 2013

Solution

A repeat dose of steroid should bring the BP up to normal levels if the cause of the hypotension is due to lack of systemic hydrocortisone.

Discussion

In a previous case of an adult patient with steroid-dependent chronic obstructive pulmonary disease, severe hypotension developed intraoperatively [1] during excision of a bladder tumor, despite an appropriate preoperative dose of hydrocortisone. The vascular collapse occurred after massive hemorrhage, even with adequate volume resuscitation. The vasoactive agent was also unsuccessful in restoring vascular tone, until a repeat dose of hydrocortisone was given. This repeat dose caused an immediate sustained improvement in arterial pressure (Fig. 9.1).

Recommendation

A repeat dose of hydrocortisone is necessary to prevent severe operative hypotension in patients recovering from chronic steroid therapy when massive blood loss ensues.

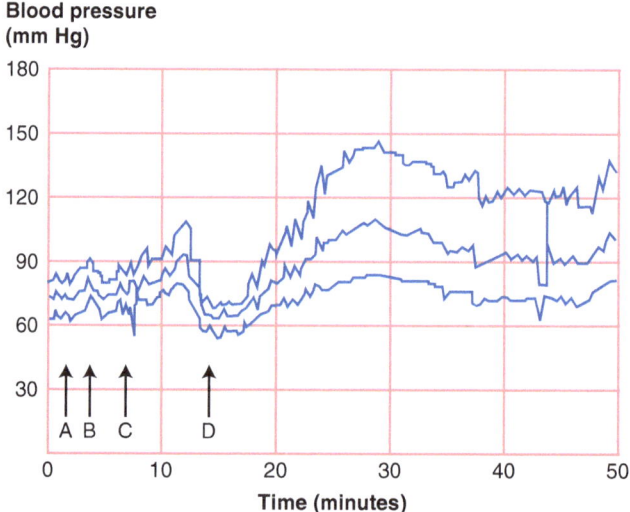

Fig. 9.1 The effect of IV hydrocortisone, 100 mg, on arterial blood pressure is shown at D. At A, B, and C, IV epinephrine boluses of 20 μg, 60 μg, and 100 μg, respectively, were administered. Prior doses of phenylephrine had no clinical effect. Reproduced with permission from Ratner EF, Allen R, Mihm FG, Brock-Utne JG. Failure of steroid supplementation to prevent operative hypotension in a patient receiving chronic steroid therapy. Anesth Analg. 1996;82:1–3

Reference

1. Ratner EF, Allen R, Mihm FG, Brock-Utne JG. Failure of steroid supplementation to prevent operative hypotension in a patient receiving chronic steroid therapy. Anesth Analg. 1996; 82:1–3.

Suggested Reading

Claussen M, Landercasper J, Cogbill T. Acute adrenal insufficiency presenting as shock after trauma and surgery: three cases and review of the literature. J Trauma. 1992;32:94–100.

Fraser CG, Preuss FS, Bigford WD. Adrenal atrophy and irreversible shock associated with cortisone therapy. JAMA. 1952;149:1542–3.

Kehlet H, Binder C. Adrenocortical function and clinical course during and after surgery in unsupplemented glucocorticoid-treated patients. Br J Anaesth. 1973;45:1043–8.

Sampson PA, Winstone NE, Brooke BN. Adrenal function in surgical patients after steroid therapy. Lancet. 1962;2:322–3.

Chapter 10
Case 10: Changing a Nasotracheal Tube for an Oral Tube in the Intensive Care Unit

A 10-year-old boy, otherwise healthy, is admitted to the trauma center after a motor vehicle accident. He has suffered a fracture of the second cervical vertebrae without neurologic deficit. The fracture is managed with the application of a halo-fixator, and he is observed in the intensive care unit (ICU). Twenty-four hours later, he develops respiratory distress and pulmonary congestion. An electrocardiogram (ECG) reveals moderate aortic valve regurgitation, probably as a result of the blunt chest trauma. A decision is made to treat the pulmonary edema with tracheal intubation and intermittent positive pressure ventilation. The halo-fixator makes direct laryngoscopy impossible. A nasal endotracheal intubation is undertaken using the fiber-optic bronchoscope, without incident.

Several days later, a diagnosis of maxillary sinusitis is made. The ICU team asks you to change the nasotracheal tube for an oral tube. How will you safely and quickly change the nasal endotracheal tube (ETT) for an oral one? To leave the nasal ETT in and discount fear of disseminated sepsis is not an option.

You discard the following options because they are considered hazardous:

1. Remove nasal ETT over bougie or tube changer followed by fiber-optic oral reintubation.
2. Pass an oral fiber-optic scope along the side of the existing nasal ETT. When the scope is safely in the trachea, remove the nasal ETT.

Question

What else can you suggest?

Solution

Pass one fiber-optic bronchoscope down the existing nasal ETT. A second fiber-optic bronchoscope directs a gum-elastic bougie along the side of the existing ETT into the trachea. The nasal fiber-optic scope confirms the correct placement of the gum-elastic bougie, the nasal ETT can be removed, and an oral tube can be placed over the bougie.

Discussion

To suggest two bronchoscopies was unheard of in the mid-1980s. Today, when most hospitals have at least three to four fiber-optic carts, such a procedure is no longer a problem. The solution, in this case, is similar to a case reported by Hambly and Field [1].

Recommendation

When faced with difficult airway problems, it is important to be creative in the interest of safety.

Reference

1. Hambly PR, Field JM. An unusual case for reintubation. Anaesthesia. 1995;50:568.

Chapter 11
Case 11: Blocked Intravenous Line During Rapid-Sequence Induction

An 8-year-old, previously healthy boy (30 kg) is scheduled for an emergency appendectomy. The patient is taken to the operating room. An intravenous (IV) line (20-gauge) in the antecubital fossa has already been started in the emergency room and is working fine. Routine monitoring equipment is placed on the child (electrocardiogram [ECG], pulse oximeter, noninvasive blood pressure [BP], and precordial stethoscope). General anesthesia is induced with thiopental (100 mg) followed by rocuronium (20 mg) with cricoid pressure. Precipitation is noted in the IV tubing. The precipitation is so severe that the IV is completely occluded. The patient is asleep, but no effect of neuromuscular relaxation, as per nerve stimulator, is seen after 90 s. You attempt laryngoscopy but fail to see the epiglottis because the child is moving his head and upper limbs. Vital signs remain stable.

Question

What will you do now?

J.G. Brock-Utne, *Near Misses in Pediatric Anesthesia*,
DOI 10.1007/978-1-4614-7040-3_11, © Springer Science+Business Media New York 2013

Solution

1. Maintain cricoid pressure.
2. Give succinylcholine under the tongue in the usual IV dose. The onset is as quick as with IV succinylcholine. Intramuscular (IM) injection of the drug could also be used, but the onset is longer than with sublingual administration. It takes at least 2 min for the full effect of IM succinylcholine to take place.

Discussion

Rocuronium has been considered an appropriate alternative to suxamethonium in certain circumstances when rapid-sequence in induction is indicated. Unfortunately, if mixing of rocuronium and thiopental does occur, a dense, white precipitate forms within the IV tubing. This precipitate has been known to cause complete obstruction of flow [1].

Recommendations

If thiopental and rocuronium are used together, as in a rapid-sequence technique, it is imperative to flush the IV thiopental with the carrier fluid before rocuronium is given. This can be done by a saline flush or by squeezing the bulb on a blood-giving set.

If one does not have a free-flowing IV, an alternative induction agent or succinylcholine should be considered.

Reference

1. Playfair PA, Uncles DR. Rocuronium and rapid sequence induction. Anaesthesia. 1995;50:663.

Chapter 12
Case 12: Postinduction Difficult Intubation

A 4-year-old, previously healthy boy is scheduled for tonsillectomy under general anesthesia. The patient is taken to the operating room, and routine monitoring equipment is placed on the child. An inhalation induction with sevoflurane is uneventful. An intravenous (IV) line is inserted, and vecuronium in a usual dose is given. RAE tubes (nasal preformed endotracheal tube [ETT]) of suitable size are not available. A (cut to size) standard uncuffed No. 5 nasal tube is inserted through the right nostril. The nasal tube is cut so that only the tube's connector is seen outside the nostril. The connector is attached to a catheter mount, placed toward the forehead, and connected to a breathing system. The child's lungs are manually ventilated. The surgeon covers the patient's head, nose, and breathing system with a "turban." Immediately thereafter the lungs become less compliant, and manual ventilation is considered very difficult. Listening to the chest confirms bilateral air entry, but breath sounds are decreased. The turban is immediately removed. This results in the immediate disappearance of the problem. A suction catheter is passed easily through the whole length of the nasal tube, and only minimal secretions are aspirated. As ventilation is now deemed to be adequate, the patient's head is redraped. However, manual ventilation again becomes difficult, and you know that if you persist with this inadequate ventilation, then desaturation, hypoxia, and so forth will result. The surgeon is not pleased and you are now wondering what to do.

J.G. Brock-Utne, *Near Misses in Pediatric Anesthesia*,
DOI 10.1007/978-1-4614-7040-3_12, © Springer Science+Business Media New York 2013

Solution

You replaced the ETT connector with a Magill's curved nasal connector and no further problems occur [1].

Discussion

It is not unusual for the weight of drapes to kink an ETT at the point where it emerges from either mouth or nose. If transparent drapes are used, the problem can quickly be detected. In this case, however, the ETT was kinked *inside* the nose by the weight of the turban. To solve this problem, the Magill connector creates a minimal gap between the breathing system and the forehead; hence, the ETT is less likely to kink. A small armored tube could be a useful alternative; however, the Magill connector is a more economical and easier solution.

Recommendation

When RAE endotracheal tubes are not available, the Magill connector is very useful to reduce the incidence of kinking of the ETT. This is especially true when the connector and breathing systems are over the forehead and covered by heavy drapes.

Reference

1. Stacy M, Asai T. Kinking of a tracheal tube in the nasal cavity. Anaesthesia. 1995;50:917.

Chapter 13
Case 13: Blunt Upper Airway Trauma in a Patient with Recent Polysubstance Abuse

An 18-year-old man is an unrestrained driver who is rear-ended. He states that he hit his neck on the steering wheel and he has difficulty in swallowing. A computed tomography (CT) scan of the neck shows a fracture of the thyroid cartilage without other evidence of significant airway injury. An emergency operative examination under general anesthesia is planned with repair of the thyroid fracture followed by tracheostomy.

Additional history reveals that the patient regularly consumes the following:

1. Up to 12 cans of beer daily (his last drink was 2 h ago).
2. Cocaine intranasally, the last time about 12 h ago.
3. Inhaled amphetamines, the last time 3 days before surgery.
4. Intravenous (IV) narcotics, the last time in the not-too-distant past.

He also smokes one pack of cigarettes daily and has mild asthma treated with inhaled beta-agonist medication.

On examination, the patient is found alert and cooperative with no apparent respiratory distress. Vital signs are blood pressure (BP) 129/71, pulse 75, respiratory rate (RR) 18, temperature 36.9 °C. He has a class 1 airway with no damaged teeth. The neck shows no gross deformity. However, swelling and tenderness are found over the right side thyroid cartilage. He exhibits no stridor or subcutaneous emphysema, no hoarseness, and no tracheal deviation. He has good cervical neck motion.

Examination of the chest reveals no other injury and clear bilateral chest sounds with normal heart tones. His hematocrit (Hct) is 45 %, and his chest X-ray is within normal limits.

Question

How would you anesthetize this patient?

J.G. Brock-Utne, *Near Misses in Pediatric Anesthesia*,   37
DOI 10.1007/978-1-4614-7040-3_13, © Springer Science+Business Media New York 2013

Solution

In this case, a tracheotomy was performed under local anesthesia. Lidocaine without epinephrine was used. A 7.0 anode tube was inserted and secured, and general anesthesia was induced with propofol and maintained with nitrous oxide in oxygen, isoflurane, and fentanyl. Panendoscopy showed moderate edema of the left and right false vocal cords, and a small hematoma of the left true vocal cord. The fracture was repaired, the anode tube was removed, and a No. 4 tracheostomy tube was inserted over a gum-elastic bougie [1]. The patient had an uneventful postoperative course and was discharged the next day.

Discussion

At least two potential anesthetic problems exist in this case:

1. *Airway*: The safest method to achieve control of the airway is to perform a tracheostomy under local anesthesia. The possibility of losing the airway during induction of general anesthesia is real, as is the chance of further damaging the thyroid cartilage. Most surgeons prefer to have no endotracheal tube (ETT) near their field. Also, the increased chance of postoperative laryngeal edema should not be forgotten.
2. *Cocaine*: Cocaine toxicity may lead to sudden death [2]. After nasal or oral ingestion, a delay of up to an hour can occur before convulsions and demise [3]. Existing heart disease is not a prerequisite for developing cardiac problems due to cocaine. The majority of deaths from cocaine are the result of deliberate or accidental overdose. The cardiac problems include vasospasm, myocardial infarction, myocarditis, cardiomyopathy, arrhythmias, and pulmonary edema [4, 5]. Neurologic problems include seizures, malignant hyperpyrexia, hypertension, encephalopathy, stroke, and respiratory arrest [6]. Other concerns include thrombocytopenia, mesenteric ischemia, and increased platelet aggregability [7]. We have described a case of preoperative marijuana inhalation causing severe uvular edema [8].

The use of lidocaine without epinephrine is more likely to be a theoretical concern than a real practical issue. In the interest of safety, however, it should be excluded. Marked hypertension and tachycardia could result from absorption of the epinephrine. Should severe hypertension result, an alpha blocker should be available. It has been suggested that beta blockade alone may worsen hypertension by unopposed alpha stimulation [9]. Calcium antagonists for arrhythmias should be considered [10].

If convulsions occur before anesthesia, then benzodiazepines or thiopental are indicated. However, control of the airway with adequate oxygenation is paramount during convulsion. Development of convulsion, in this case, could have proved to be a serious problem because of the patient's airway.

Recommendation

Although this patient's airway was class 1, the safest anesthetic technique for this patient is a tracheostomy under local anesthesia followed by general anesthesia.

References

1. Robles B, Hester J, Brock-Utne JG. Remember the gum-elastic bougie at extubation. J Clin Anesth. 1993;5:329–31.
2. Fleming JA, Byck R, Garash PG. Pharmacology and therapeutic applications of cocaine. Anesthesiology. 1990;73:518–31.
3. Isner JM, Estes 3rd NA, Thompson PD, Costanzo-Nordin MR, Subramanian R, Miller G, et al. Acute cardiac events temporally related to cocaine abuse. N Engl J Med. 1986;315:1438–43.
4. Isner JM, Chokshi SK. Cardiac complications of cocaine abuse. Annu Rev Med. 1991;42:133–8.
5. Minor RL, Scott BD, Brown DD, Winniford MD. Cocaine-induced myocardial infarction in patients with normal coronary arteries. Ann Intern Med. 1991;115:797–806.
6. Sauer C. Recurrent embolic stroke and cocaine-related cardiomyopathy. Stroke. 1991;22: 1203–5.
7. Orser B. Thrombocytopenia and cocaine abuse. Anesthesiology. 1991;74:195–6.
8. Mallet AM, Roberson T, Brock-Utne JG. Preoperative marijuana inhalation—an airway concern. Can J Anaesth. 1996;43:691–3.
9. Gay GR, Loper KA. Control of cocaine induced hypertension with labetalol. Anesth Analg. 1988;67:92.
10. Cregler LL, Mark H. Medical complications of cocaine abuse. N Engl J Med. 1986;315: 1495–500.

Chapter 14
Case 14: The Stuck Elevator

A 6-year-old girl falls out of a car (traveling 35 mph) onto her left side. She is taken to the hospital with C-spine precautions. On arrival, the patient is alert and oriented. The C-spine films are negative. The patient is hemodynamically stable in the emergency room without evidence of external injuries other than superficial abrasion. She has no long-bone fractures, and two peripheral (18-gauge) intravenous (IV) lines are inserted. Her hematocrit (Hct) is 30 %. Just as she is about to be discharged she complains of abdominal pain. An abdominal computed tomography (CT) scan reveals intraperitoneal fluid and a ruptured splenic capsule. The patient is scheduled for an emergency laparotomy and transported to the operating room with oxygen, 6 l per minute, breathing spontaneously with a mask airway. A Jackson Rees modification of the Ayres T-piece is used to provide oxygen. In the elevator, the patient complains of sudden onset of chest pain and difficulty in breathing.

At that point, the elevator stops between two floors. You do the following:

1. Press the alarm bell in the elevator.
2. Examine the patient. No cyanosis is seen (as far as you can tell in the artificial light—you have no oximeter with you). There is minimal air entry bilaterally but no adventitious sounds.
3. The patient feels she is not getting enough air. You attempt to assist ventilation with your mask airway using the Jackson Rees modification of the Ayres T-piece, only to discover that your collapsible ventilation bag has a large hole in it and is therefore useless. You have no drugs, laryngoscope, endotracheal tubes (ETTs), or self-inflating (Ambu) bags.

Question

What will you do to try to assist ventilation in this patient without resorting to mouth-to-mouth resuscitation?

J.G. Brock-Utne, *Near Misses in Pediatric Anesthesia*,
DOI 10.1007/978-1-4614-7040-3_14, © Springer Science+Business Media New York 2013

Solution

1. Reassure the patient.
2. Take the damaged collapsible bag off and intermittently occlude the corrugated tubing of the Jackson Rees modification (Fig. 14.1).
3. Help her sit up in the bed.

Discussion

The chest pain and the shortness of breath were believed to be secondary to intra-abdominal blood with diaphragmatic referral. By sitting the patient up, the symptoms improved, and by the time the elevator was operational again (10 min), the patient did not complain of pain. The patient made an uneventful recovery from her ruptured spleen.

Recommendation

During transport of potentially problematic patients, it is essential that emergency drugs, ETTs, oxygen supply, a Jackson Rees modification (Mapleson F), and an oximeter are readily available.

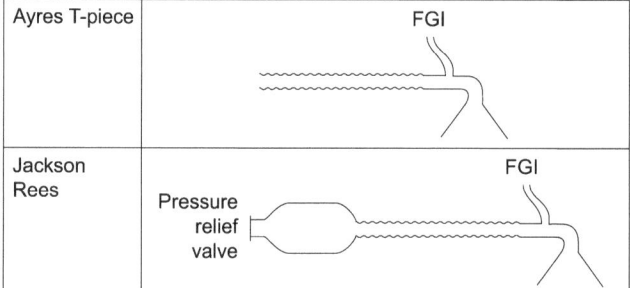

Fig. 14.1 Ayres T-piece (Mapleson E) is shown without a collapsible bag as it was originally described. Ayres ventilated the children by occluding, with his thumb, the distal end of the corrugated tubing (exhalation tube) and watching the chest exertions. Jackson Rees modified the Ayres T-piece by placing a collapsible bag with a pressure relief valve at its end. This system is now also known as a Mapleson F. Although it is difficult to scavenge from a Mapleson E, it is easier with a Mapleson F (*FGI* fresh gas intake)

Chapter 15
Case 15: Postoperative Upper Airway Obstruction

A 16-year-old boy (80 kg) is scheduled for outpatient arthroscopy of his left knee. He is classified as an American Society of Anesthesiologists physical status I (ASA 1) and has no significant medical history. He takes no medication or illicit drugs. He is a high school wrestling champion. In the preoperative area, an intravenous (IV) infusion is started and midazolam, 1 mg, is given as a premedicant. In the operating room, his vital signs are heart rate 64 regular, blood pressure (BP) 130/70, respiratory rate (RR) 12; his chest is clear. After preoxygenation, anesthesia is induced with propofol, 150 mg, and a laryngeal mask airway (LMA) is inserted atraumatically. The surgical procedure is uneventful. On awakening from the anesthetic, the patient coughs violently and develops laryngospasm. Oxygen saturation falls below 80 %. Positive pressure mask ventilation with 100 % oxygen breaks the laryngospasm after a few minutes, but a few minutes after that, he is unable to get sufficient air into his lungs. Vital signs are normal, but the oxygen saturation is 92 % on 100 % FIO_2 via a Jackson Rees modification of the Ayres T-piece (see Chapter 14). Examination of the chest reveals bilateral crepitations all over his lung fields, and now he is coughing up pink frothy sputum.

Question

What is the cause of the problem and what will you do?

J.G. Brock-Utne, *Near Misses in Pediatric Anesthesia*,
DOI 10.1007/978-1-4614-7040-3_15, © Springer Science+Business Media New York 2013

Solution

A chest X-ray showed pulmonary edema and you gave furosemide, 20 mg. There was rapid clinical improvement. The electrocardiogram (ECG) was normal. The patient was admitted overnight for observation and discharged the next day.

Discussion

This is a classic case of negative pressure pulmonary edema (NPPE), which was first described by Oswalt et al. [1]. NPPE is a rare form of noncardiogenic pulmonary edema that may complicate upper airway obstruction [2]. It has been described as having two components. First, forceful inspiratory efforts against an obstruction may cause capillary damage. This mechanism is akin to that of re-expansion pulmonary edema [3] and creates a large transpulmonary pressure gradient favoring transudation of fluid from the pulmonary capillaries into the alveoli. Resultant hypoxia and sympathetic discharge induce vasoconstriction [4], increasing the pulmonary filtration pressure and thereby worsening the pulmonary edema. Second, NPPE usually occurs after the relief of the airway obstruction. Expiration against the obstruction creates an "auto-PEEP" (positive end-expiratory pressure) effect, preventing pulmonary flooding [5]. When the obstruction is removed, this protective effect is lost and pulmonary edema results. However, NPPE is usually self-limiting, resolving within 12–24 h of supportive therapy.

The main differential diagnosis is pulmonary aspiration; however, improvement in clinical symptoms after the correction of an airway obstruction merits the diagnosis of NPPE.

Recommendation

NPPE is uncommon, but awareness of this complication allows for early recognition and prompt treatment. Although more common in strong, healthy adults [6–8], it has also been reported in infants [9].

References

1. Oswalt CE, Gates GA, Holmstrom F. Pulmonary edema as a complication of acute airway obstruction. JAMA. 1977;238:1833–5.
2. Travis KW, Todres ID, Shannon DC. Pulmonary edema associated with croup and epiglottitis. Pediatrics. 1977;59:695–8.
3. Pavlin DJ, Nessly ML, Cheney FW. Increased pulmonary vascular permeability as a cause of re-expansion edema in rabbits. Am Rev Respir Dis. 1981;124:422–7.

4. Theodore J, Robin ED. Pathogenesis of neurogenic pulmonary edema. Lancet. 1975;2:749.
5. Pepe PE, Mariani JJ. Occult positive end-expiratory pressure in mechanically ventilated patients with air flow obstructions: the auto-peep effect. Am Rev Respir Dis. 1982;126:1666–70.
6. Cochran M, DeBattista C, Schmiesing C, Brock-Utne JG. Negative pressure pulmonary edema (a potential hazard in patients undergoing ECT). J ECT. 1999;15:168–79.
7. Homes JR, Henninger RN, Wojtys EW. Postoperative pulmonary edema in young athletic adults. Am J Sports Med. 1991;19:365–71.
8. Barin ES, Stevenson IF, Donnelly GL. Pulmonary oedema following acute upper airway obstruction. Anaesth Intensive Care. 1986;15:54–7.
9. Warner LO, Martin D, Davidson PJ, Beach TP. Negative pressure pulmonary edema, a potential hazard of muscle relaxants in awake infants. Can Anaesth J. 1990;37:580–3.

Chapter 16
Case 16: Postoperative Respiratory Complications in a Neonate

A 3-day-old boy is scheduled for repair of a tracheoesophageal fistula. No other abnormalities are noted. Anesthesia is induced with sevoflurane, and suxamethonium is given to place an endotracheal tube (ETT) (3 mm) in the trachea. Anesthesia is maintained with 70 % nitrous oxide in oxygen and halothane. Vecuronium is given as a muscle relaxant. A thoracic epidural is inserted via the caudal canal to approximately T6 [1]. During the operation, the catheter is infused with bupivacaine 0.125 % at a rate of 0.5 ml per hour. The operation is completed uneventfully, and the ETT is removed from the baby's trachea. During the first 24 h, the baby's vital signs are stable. The surgeon is keen to remove the epidural catheter and start the child on oral/rectal nonsteroidal anti-inflammatory drugs (NSAIDs). You agree but leave the epidural catheter in situ. After 2 h, the respiratory rate increases from 45 to 55 breaths per minute. The baby's saturation decreases from 95 % to 90 %. The inspired oxygen is increased to 30 % and more rectal analgesic is administered. Continuous positive airway pressure (CPAP) (5 cm H_2O) is given, and some improvement is seen in the vital signs. You feel happier about the baby until the nurse brings you a chest X-ray of the patient taken 5 min previously. This shows a right middle and lower lobe collapse. The oxygen saturation is now 88 %.

Questions

Will you wait and see, or will you do something? If so, what will you do?

Solution

The epidural infusion was restarted with bupivacaine. After 5–10 min, the vital signs improved significantly. The baby continued to receive the epidural infusion up to 40 h postoperatively and after that made an uneventful recovery.

Discussion

Before 1975, very few pediatric patients received regional anesthesia for intraoperative or postoperative pain relief. Since then, there has been great interest in this field and much has been learned [2, 3]. Perioperative epidural bupivacaine has been shown to attenuate the stress response to surgery better than do systemic opioids [4].

In this case, the too-early termination of an adequate epidural anesthetic and replacement with an inferior analgesic led to pain, splinting of the rib cage, and collapse of the lung. This case is similar to a previous report [5].

Recommendation

When a call is made to remove an adequate epidural, it is prudent to leave the epidural in situ until alternate analgesics are seen to work satisfactorily. To do otherwise can, in certain cases, lead to serious clinical problems [5].

References

1. Bosenberg AT, Bland BAR, Schulte-Steinberg O, Downing JW. Thoracic epidural anaesthesia via the caudal route in infants. Anesthesiology. 1988;69:365–9.
2. Berde C. Regional anesthesia in children: what have we learned? Anesth Analg. 1996;83: 897–900.
3. Giaufre E, Dalens B, Gombert A. Epidemiology and morbidity of regional anesthesia in children: a one-year prospective survey of the French-language society of pediatric anesthesiologists. Anesth Analg. 1996;83:904–12.
4. Rowe P, Simon L. Effect of extradural analgesia on stress responses to abdominal surgery in infants. Br J Anaesth. 1993;70:654–60.
5. Cass LJ, Howard RF. Respiratory complications due to inadequate analgesia following thoracotomy in a neonate. Anaesthesia. 1994;49:879–80.

Chapter 17
Case 17: Pregnant Teenager with a Bad Outcome

A 17-year-old primigravida (85 kg) is admitted to the hospital at 7 p.m. She is 39 weeks pregnant and in labor. Fetal distress is diagnosed and an emergency cesarean section is scheduled. The patient refuses both spinal and epidural anesthesia. She is taken to operating room No. 4 and routine monitors are placed. She is very nervous and does not want the oxygen mask for preoxygenation. You anesthetize her with a rapid-sequence technique consisting of metoclopramide; an antacid, 30 ml per os; etomidate, 18 mg; and succinylcholine, 100 mg, with cricoid pressure. After the endotracheal tube (ETT) is placed in the trachea, anesthesia is maintained with 50 % nitrous oxide in oxygen with isoflurane 0.8 %. Further muscle relaxation is provided by intravenous (IV) injection of vecuronium, 7 mg. At delivery, the child cries immediately and has an Apgar score of 8/8 at 1 min after delivery. After delivery of the infant, the mother receives morphine, 10 mg IV, and the nitrous oxide is increased to 70 % in oxygen. At the end of the surgery, the isoflurane is turned off. The residual effect of the nondepolarizing drug is antagonized with neostigmine, 5 mg, mixed with atropine, 1.2 mg, IV. The patient starts to breathe spontaneously. The nitrous oxide is turned off and 100 % oxygen is given. Three to four minutes later, the oxygen saturation alarms. The saturation is now 88 %, down from 100 %. You check the monitor but it seems to be working as the heart rate per the oximeter and electrocardiogram (ECG) is identical at 100 beats per minute (bpm) up from 82 bpm. You examine your patient and discover that she is cyanosed and, despite all attempts to resuscitate her, she is declared dead 20 min later. You and the whole team are devastated.

Question

What could have gone wrong?

J.G. Brock-Utne, *Near Misses in Pediatric Anesthesia*,
DOI 10.1007/978-1-4614-7040-3_17, © Springer Science+Business Media New York 2013

Solution

This tragic case happened to a friend of mine. A maintenance crew had worked on the oxygen and nitrous oxide pipelines supplying operating room No. 4 that afternoon, from 5 to 6 p.m. This event was unknown to the operating room staff at 7:10 p.m., when the pregnant teenager was wheeled into the operating room. Unfortunately, the workers had switched the pipes so that nitrous oxide was oxygen and oxygen was nitrous oxide. The lack of preoxygenation in this case precluded the anesthesiologist making the diagnosis. Adding to the anesthesiologist's problems was the fact that the oxygen analyzer was later found to be defective.

Later that night, a small child was admitted in respiratory distress to the same hospital. The mother thought a peanut was lodged in the trachea. The child was taken to operating room No. 4. When another anesthesiologist attempted to induce the child with 100 % oxygen (which was actually 100 % nitrous oxide), the child quickly desaturated. The anesthesiologist decided to try another machine in another operating room. Here, induction with 100 % oxygen was uneventful and the peanut was successfully removed. Operating room No. 4 was closed. The next morning the room was inspected and the fault found.

Recommendations

There are two good reasons for preoxygenating any patient:

1. To increase the oxygen reserve.
2. To make certain that the gas labeled "oxygen" actually is oxygen. If it is 100 % nitrous oxide, you will soon find out.

Chapter 18
Case 18: Tension Pneumoperitoneum

A 16-year-old girl is admitted to the hospital with increasing abdominal pain. Her history is unremarkable and she is on no treatment. A diagnosis of a perforated viscous is made. Abdominal X-rays show a large pneumoperitoneum with elevation of the diaphragm. She is transferred to the operating room with a 4-l oxygen mask for an emergency laparotomy. She is unable to lie flat because of her respiratory distress. Her vital signs include a sinus tachycardia of 110 beats per minute (bpm), blood pressure (BP) 150/90, respiration shallow with a rate of 32, and oxygen saturation 95 %. She complains of severe abdominal pain, cannot get enough air, and is very worried.

Question

How will you anesthetize this patient, who should be treated as a full stomach?

J.G. Brock-Utne, *Near Misses in Pediatric Anesthesia*,
DOI 10.1007/978-1-4614-7040-3_18, © Springer Science+Business Media New York 2013

Solution

You can either (1) do a tracheal intubation with the patient in the sitting position using a fiber-optic laryngoscope or (2) do a rapid-sequence induction.

Fiber-Optic Laryngoscope

Intragastric pressures measured in normal fasting adult patients may reach 30 cm H_2O [1, 2]. The distance between the lower esophageal sphincter (LES) and the upper esophageal sphincter exceeds 25 cm in most adults. Hence, even if the LES provides little resistance to the efflux of gastric content, it is considered unlikely that normal intragastric pressure, responsible for passive regurgitation, would be sufficient to force the gastric contents into the oropharynx in a patient sitting fully upright. Before securing the airway fiber-optically, it is imperative to decrease gastric volume and acidity and increase LES tone [2–7]. Adequate topical anesthesia should be provided, preferably with the atomizer (Magill spray), using a combination of lidocaine 4 % (8 ml), tetracaine 20 % (2 ml), and cocaine 2 % (2 ml). If the patient can tolerate it, 2 ml of the aforementioned mixture can be injected through the cricothyroid membrane to provide intratracheal anesthesia. Thereafter, a standard oral fiber-optic intubation can be performed.

It is important to remember that topical anesthesia abolishes the laryngeal protective reflexes.

Rapid-Sequence Induction

1. Intravenous (IV) sedation (if considered safe).
2. A 60 % head-up tilt.
3. Preoxygenation.
4. Several floor lifts for the anesthesiologist to be able to stand sufficiently tall to visualize the vocal cords and therefore intubate the trachea safely.
5. IV induction with ketamine.
6. Cricoid pressure. This may be one of the drawbacks of a rapid-sequence induction in this position because anesthesiologists have problems with its safe and efficient application even with the patient supine [8–10]. One should also consider the possibility of carotid body stimulation.
7. No nitrous oxide, at least before the pneumoperitoneum tension is released.
8. Be prepared for a potential associated pneumothorax (see Chap. 20).

Discussion

At laparotomy, a perforated gastric ulcer is found and repaired. The development of the tension pneumoperitoneum is thought to be caused by a flaplike mechanism fed by aerophagy. Pneumoperitoneum is caused in 90 % of cases by perforation of an intestinal viscus and in 10 % by pulmonary barotrauma. In one adult case, fatal tension pneumoperitoneum with associated pneumothorax was reported [11].

Recommendation

In these cases, securing the airway with a fiber-optic technique may be the safest solution.

References

1. Dow TGB, Chamney AR, Wraight WJ, Simons RS. The application of cricoid pressure: an assessment and a survey of its practice. Anaesthesia. 1983;38:457–60.
2. Brock-Utne JG, Dow TG, Welman S, Dimopoulos GE, Moshal MG. The effect of metoclopramide on the lower oesophageal sphincter in late pregnancy. Anaesth Intensive Care. 1978;6:26–9.
3. Andrews AD, Brock-Utne JG, Downing JW. Protection against pulmonary acid aspiration with ranitidine. Anaesthesia. 1982;37:22–5.
4. Brock-Utne JG, Downing JW, Humphrey D. Effect of ranitidine given before atropine sulphate on lower esophageal sphincter tone. Anaesth Intensive Care. 1984;12:140–2.
5. Brock-Utne JG. Domperidone antagonizes the relaxant effect of atropine on the lower esophageal sphincter. Anesth Analg. 1980;59:921–4.
6. Howard FA, Sharp DS. Effects of metoclopramide on gastric emptying during labour. BMJ. 1973;1:446–8.
7. Murphy DF, Nally B, Gardiner J. Effect of metoclopramide on gastric emptying before elective emergency caesarean section. Br J Anaesth. 1984;56:1113–6.
8. Raidoo DM, Rocke DA, Brock-Utne JG, Marszalek A, Engelbrecht HE. Critical volume for pulmonary aspiration. Reappraisal in a primate model. Br J Anaesth. 1990;65:248–50.
9. Howells THE, Chamney AR, Wraight WJ, Simons RS. The application of cricoid pressure: an assessment and a survey of its practice. Anaesthesia. 1983;38:457–60.
10. Wraight WJ, Chamney AR, Howells THE. The determination of an effective cricoid pressure. Anaesthesia. 1983;38:461–6.
11. Critchley LAH, Rowbottom S. Fatal tension pneumoperitoneum with pneumothorax. Anaesth Intensive Care. 1994;22:298–9.

Chapter 19
Case 19: A Patient with Status Asthmaticus

An 8-year-old girl presents to the emergency room with exacerbation of her asthma. She has been hospitalized five times previously, requiring salbutamol via nebulizer, oral slow-release theophylline preparation, and chest physiotherapy. She presents now with increased shortness of breath and wheezing that has gradually worsened over the past 24 h. On examination, she is pale, distressed, and hardly able to speak. Her vital signs are the following: heart rate: 136 beats per minute (bpm); blood pressure (BP): 140/60; and respiratory rate: 30 breaths per minute with poor air entry to both lung fields and soft, high-pitched wheezes heard all over.

The initial management includes oxygen via mask at 10 l per minute, salbutamol 0.5 % via nebulizer, aminophylline via intravenous (IV) infusion, and a bolus dose of hydrocortisone, 250 mg IV. Initial blood gas shows a pH of 7.31, PCO_2 of 50 mmHg, and PO_2 of 77 mmHg. The patient does not respond to the therapy and appears tired and listless. A repeat blood gas shows the PCO_2 has risen to 90 mmHg. A decision to mechanically ventilate the patient is made. An awake blind nasotracheal technique is used. The tube is passed with some difficulty through the right nostril but readily enters the trachea. The patient is sedated with morphine and midazolam. Vecuronium is given for muscle relaxation. The nasotracheal intubation is complicated by a moderately severe epistaxis requiring nasal and oral packing, with good effect. However, the peak airway pressure is higher than 100 cm H_2O, and it is difficult to ventilate the patient's lungs by hand because the chest is found to be very "tight." There are audible wheezes bilaterally. A chest X-ray confirms the correct placement of the endotracheal tube (ETT), and no evidence of pneumothorax is found. Salbutamol is administered continuously via nebulizer and infused by IV, together with aminophylline. Epinephrine, 1 ml (1:10,000), is administered via the nasotracheal tube. The above treatment elicits very little improvement in peak airway pressures. An arterial blood gas reveals pH of 7.10, PCO_2 of 96 mmHg, and PO_2 of 200 mmHg.

Question

Besides trying other drugs, what will you do now?

Solution

A tracheal suction catheter should always be passed in these cases to assess patency of the ETT. The catheter meets with serious obstruction at what is perceived to be the distal end of the ETT. Firm pressure is applied to the catheter and the obstruction is eliminated. The suction catheter is removed with some blood seen in the catheter. Immediately thereafter, the peak inspiratory pressures fall to high-normal levels, and the arterial blood gas shows improvement.

Discussion

Magill [1] described the technique of blind nasotracheal intubation in an awake patient. This is considerably safer than endotracheal intubation after sedation and muscle relaxation in many of the aforementioned cases. Hypoxia, caused by inadvertent esophageal intubation or prolonged and difficult endotracheal intubation, together with the potential for aspiration of gastric content, is inherent with the use of the sedation and muscle relaxation. However, complications of the Magill technique are also well documented [2–5]. Epistaxis is seen in up to 13 % of cases [3]. Obstruction of the ETT by sputum plugs [6], blood clots [7], dried lubricant jelly [8], inferior [9] and middle [10] turbinates, and nasal polyp [11] are well described.

The case reported here is similar to a previous report [12], in which a turbinate was dislodged from the tip of the ETT to the right main bronchus after the passing of the suction catheter. The turbinate later led to a right lung collapse, which was resolved after the removal of the turbinate at bronchoscopy. Another case report [9] mentioned the avulsion of an inferior turbinate during blind nasal intubation in which the subsequent obstruction of the ETT led to the sudden appearance of bronchospasm.

Recommendation

During blind nasal intubation, partial or total obstruction of the ETT can occur—a fact that can easily be forgotten during the often highly charged treatment of an asthmatic. One automatically could assume that the increased peak pressures and audible wheeze are due solely to the asthma and not due in whole or in part to an obstructed ETT.

To prevent the avulsion or impaction of material at the tip of the ETT during the passage through the nose, a Foley catheter has been suggested for use as an obturator [11].

References

1. Magill W. Lest we forget. Anesthesia. 1975;30:476–90.
2. Blanc VF, Tremblay NA. The complications of tracheal intubation: a new classification and a review of the literature. Anesth Analg. 1974;53:202.
3. Iserson KV. Blind nasotracheal intubation. Ann Emerg Med. 1981;10:468–71.
4. Tintinalli JE, Claffy J. Complications of nasotracheal intubation. Ann Emerg Med. 1981;10: 142–4.
5. Danzl DF, Thomas DM. Nasotracheal intubations in the emergency department. Crit Care Med. 1980;8:677–82.
6. Cohen IL, Weinberg RF, Fein IA, Rowinski GS. Endotracheal tube occlusion associated with the use of heat and moisture exchanges in the intensive care unit. Crit Care Med. 1988;16: 277–9.
7. Heinzig D, Rosenblatt R. Thrombotic occlusion of nasotracheal tube. Anesthesiology. 1979; 51:484–6.
8. Veihra A, Tanaka A, Oda M, Sato T. Obstruction of an endotracheal tube by lidocaine jelly. Anesthesiology. 1981;55:598–9.
9. Boysen K. An unusual case of nasotracheal tube occlusion [letter]. Anesthesia. 1985;40:1024.
10. Scamman FL, Sabin RW. An unusual complication of nasotracheal intubation. Anesthesiology. 1983;59:352–3.
11. Kawamoto M, Shimudzu Y. A balloon catheter for nasal intubation. Anesthesiology. 1983; 59:484.
12. Bernard SA, Jones B, Mac C. Endotracheal tube obstruction in a patient with status asthmaticus. Anaesth Intensive Care. 1991;19:121–3.

Chapter 20
Case 20: Intraoperative Decrease in Electrocardiogram Amplitude: Cause for Concern?

A 3-year-old boy (28 lb) is scheduled for a left nephrectomy for a Wilms' tumor. His medical history is unremarkable except for hematuria and an abdominal mass. The patient has no known drug allergies, and the family history is negative for anesthesia-related problems.

General anesthesia is induced via face mask with sevoflurane 1–4 % in nitrous oxide 70 % and 30 % oxygen after all necessary noninvasive monitoring equipment is placed on the child. After the child is asleep, an intravenous (IV) line is inserted and 2 mg vecuronium is administered to facilitate tracheal intubation. Ninety minutes into the operation, the lead II electrocardiogram (ECG) tracing is noted to be dramatically reduced in amplitude when compared to the preinduction tracing (Fig. 20.1). The heart rate, blood pressure (BP), end-tidal CO_2, and airway pressures have not changed. Breath sounds continue to be equal bilaterally.

Questions

Are you concerned? If so, what could the problem be?

J.G. Brock-Utne, *Near Misses in Pediatric Anesthesia*,   59
DOI 10.1007/978-1-4614-7040-3_20, © Springer Science+Business Media New York 2013

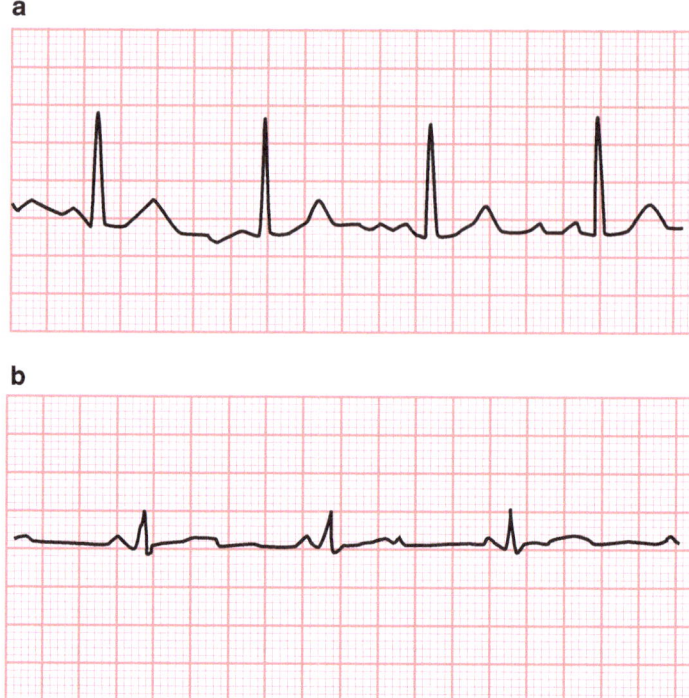

Fig. 20.1 (**a**) The electrocardiogram (ECG) before induction of anesthesia. (**b**) The ECG after nephrectomy. Reproduced with permission Botz G, Brock-Utne JG. Are electrocardiogram changes the first sign of impending peri-operative pneumothorax? Anesthesia. 1992;47:1057–9

Solution

You are concerned because you think a possible pneumothorax is developing.

1. You change the anesthetic gases from 70 % nitrous oxide in oxygen to 100 % oxygen with sevoflurane 1–2 %.
2. A portable chest X-ray is requested.
3. A chest drain should be made available. An emergency chest drain can be made from available anesthesia equipment within a minute should the need arise [1].

Discussion

Decreased ECG amplitude produced by spontaneous pneumothoraces has been described as a diagnostic aid in the awake breathing patient [2–4]. In our case [5], after having diagnosed a pneumothorax, we elected not to put in a chest drain

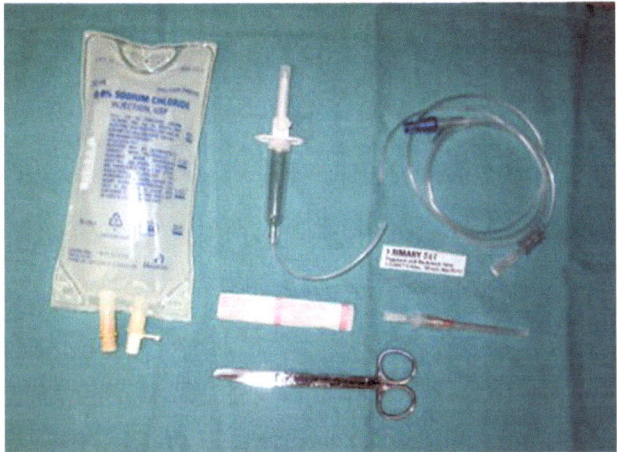

Fig. 20.2 The equipment necessary for the rapid construction of an underwater seal apparatus includes the following: one 250 ml glass or plastic container of IV fluid, a primary IV set, scissor, IV 14-gauge catheter, and an 18-gauge or larger needle. The method includes cutting the primary IV set in half as shown in the figure. The piercing pin of the primary IV set (*on the left*) is inserted into the IV plastic container after having removed the white stopper. The other cut end of the primary IV set (*on the right*) is inserted into the outlet of the 250 ml plastic container. This is the outlet that has been pierced with the pin of the primary IV set. The end of the primary IV tubing is introduced well below the fluid level. The 14-gauge IV catheter is inserted into the pleural cavity on the affected side through the second intercostal space in the mid-clavicular line. The proximal end of the 14-gauge catheter is then attached to the male adapter on the primary IV. The other end of this primary IV set that is attached to the male adapter is in the 250 ml container. The large bore needle (>18-gauge) is inserted through the medication injection port of the plastic container to act as a vent

immediately because the patient's general condition remained stable. However, 25 min later, without any further change in the amplitude of the ECG, there was a sudden decrease in oxygen saturation to less than 95 %. The mean arterial pressure decreased to 40 mmHg and peak inspiratory pressure rose from 25 to 58 cm H_2O. Decreased air entry was noted on the left. The chest drain had not yet arrived so the emergency chest drain (Fig. 20.2) was used [1]. After the placement of the chest drain, the ECG amplitude reverted to baseline levels. The patient made an uneventful recovery and was discharged 1 week later.

A right-sided intraoperative pneumothorax may not show such a dramatic decrease in amplitude for obvious reasons [6].

Recommendation

Intraoperative decreased ECG amplitude should be taken seriously [5–7].

References

1. Brock-Utne JG, Brodsky JB, Haddow G, Mark JB. A simple underwater seal apparatus for use in emergencies. J Cardiothorac Vasc Anesth. 1991;5:195–7.
2. Marten AM. The electrocardiographic changes in pneumothorax in which the heart has been rotated: the similarity of some of these changes to those indicating myocardial involvement. Am Heart J. 1928;3:472.
3. Armen RN. Frand. TV. Electrocardiographic patterns in pneumothorax. Dis Chest. 1949;15:709–10.
4. Copeland RB, Omenn GS. Electrocardiogram changes suggestive of coronary artery disease in pneumothorax. Their reversibility with upright posture. Arch Intern Med. 1970;125:151–3.
5. Botz G, Brock-Utne JG. Are electrocardiogram changes the first sign of impending peri-operative pneumothorax? Anaesthesia. 1992;47:1057–9.
6. Brock-Utne JG, Botz G. Are electrocardiograms changes the first sign of impending periopera-tive pneumothorax? Anaesthesia. 1993;48:543–4.
7. Ruo W, Rupani G. Left tension pneumothorax mimicking myocardial ischemia after percutane-ous central venous cannulation. Anesthesiology. 1992;76:306–8.

Chapter 21
Case 21: Potential Disaster: An Intravenous Line That Stops Working in the Perioperative Phase

A 10-year-old boy (30 lb) is scheduled for a left hernia repair. His medical history is otherwise unremarkable. The patient has no known drug allergies, and the family history is negative for anesthesia-related problems. An intravenous (IV) line (20 gauge) in the back of the hand is seen to be adequate; it was placed by the pediatric resident for preoperative IV antibiotic. The patient is taken to the operating room, and monitoring equipment is placed on the child (electrocardiogram [ECG], pulse oximeter, a nerve stimulator, noninvasive blood pressure [BP], and precordial stethoscope). General anesthesia is induced with propofol, 75 mg, and the patient falls asleep. The patient is easily ventilated via a face mask with sevoflurane 1–4 % with 100 % oxygen, and vecuronium, 4 mg, is given by the 20 gauge IV. After 3 min, the nerve stimulator indicates that the patient is not adequately relaxed. The IV is checked and found to be nonfunctioning. A new IV is inserted and a repeat dose of vecuronium is administered. Within 3 min, the patient is adequately relaxed, and an endotracheal tube (ETT) is inserted into the trachea atraumatically. Breath sounds are equal bilaterally. Anesthesia is maintained with nitrous oxide 70 % in oxygen with isoflurane 0.6 % and with meperidine, 15 mg. The surgery commences and concludes uneventfully. At the end of the surgery, with the patient breathing spontaneously, the ETT is removed from the patient's trachea. The child is taken to the postanesthesia care unit (PACU) asleep but arousable. Twenty minutes later, when you are about to induce anesthesia in your next case, you get a call from the PACU. You are told that your previous patient is not breathing and the oxygen saturation is now 76 %. You tell the nurse to commence artificial ventilation and you run to the PACU. In the PACU, the nurse is successfully administering oxygen 100 % via a face mask using a Jackson Rees modification of the Ayres T-piece. The oxygen saturation is now 96 %, and his vital signs include a heart rate of 140 beats per minute (bpm) and a BP of 80/50 mmHg.

Question

What will you do and what could be the cause of the respiratory arrest?

J.G. Brock-Utne, *Near Misses in Pediatric Anesthesia*,
DOI 10.1007/978-1-4614-7040-3_21, © Springer Science+Business Media New York 2013

Solution

You go to the head of the bed and reintubate the child. Vital signs continue to be normal. You note that the IV that had failed in the operating room now seems to be working. The nurse informs you that she has managed to get it to work. A nerve stimulator shows that the child is completely relaxed. The cause of the respiratory failure was most likely the vecuronium that remained in the original IV. This drug got into the systemic circulation when the nurse flushed the IV to get it working again.

Discussion

An intraoperative malfunctioning or nonfunctioning IV is not an uncommon problem. Although the aforementioned case is unusual, other intraoperative problems can also occur. At times during surgery, when the IV insertion into the vein is hidden from view, it is impossible to see if the IV is infiltrating. I have seen a case of a 60-year-old man who had to have his left arm amputated after a 4-h routine coronary artery bypass operation because of excessive IV infiltration. I have also seen a hidden IV unintentionally severed by a surgeon [1]. This led to a near disaster. If I cannot fully see the catheter, where it enters the vein, I will not use it unless absolutely necessary. If I must use it, I regularly check it for patency.

Recommendation

From the case presented, it would seem prudent to remove immediately any IV that is deemed nonfunctioning. This should prevent a potentially serious mishap.

Reference

1. Kim A, Brock-Utne JG. Another potential problem with the "hidden IV". Can J Anaesth. 1998;45:495–6.

Chapter 22
Case 22: Ventilatory Management in Major Thoracic Incisional Injury

A 17-year-old boy is admitted to the emergency room after a single 30-cm machete injury to his right chest. The incision extends from the right of the sternum at the level of T6 toward the midaxillary line. He states he had previously been in good health and is on no medical treatment. On examination, he is fully conscious, vital signs are stable, and the hematocrit (Hct) is 30 %. An intravenous (IV) line is started and an intercostal chest drain inserted. The latter is seen to be working well, but a great deal of white-pink froth is noted in the underwater seal bottle. The patient is taken to the operating room for exploration of the chest.

Questions

How would you anesthetize this patient? Would you consider using a double-lumen tube? If so, why?

J.G. Brock-Utne, *Near Misses in Pediatric Anesthesia*,   65
DOI 10.1007/978-1-4614-7040-3_22, © Springer Science+Business Media New York 2013

Solution

In this case, a rapid-sequence technique was used with cricoid pressure, and a left double-lumen tube passed easily into the trachea. Initially, both lungs were ventilated, but the patient suddenly became cyanotic with an unrecordable oxygen saturation. The right lumen of the double-lumen tube ventilating the right lung was occluded by a clamp at the mouth end, leaving only the left lung to be ventilated. The patient's color immediately improved, and the oxygen saturation rose above 97 %. A large single laceration of the lung, a 15-cm laceration of the diaphragm, and a 5-cm laceration of the liver were found. The diaphragm and the liver lacerations were repaired. The chest was closed. The right lung was seen to expand adequately, but again, when both lungs were ventilated, the oxygen saturation fell. The patient's left lung was ventilated for the next 10 h, and his vital signs remained stable. When he was able to ventilate spontaneously with both lungs via the double-lumen tube, it was removed. He continued to improve and was discharged 4 days later.

Discussion

A double-lumen tube was used in this case because of the clinical suspicion of a bronchopleural fistula. Had a single-lumen tube been used, a potential disaster could have occurred due to an inability to isolate the right lung quickly. If the injury had been to the left side, one could have placed the single lumen tube into the right main stem.

The use of a double-lumen tube in a rapid-sequence technique in patients with airway classes 1 and 2 should not be an added hazard to getting control of the airway. I have used the double-lumen tube many times in similar situations with no adverse effect. It is, however, important to have at least two smaller double-tube versions in the room. The verification of the correct position of the tube can be done either with the Brodsky technique [1] or by using fiber-optic laryngoscopy [2]. This case is similar to a previously reported incident [3]. In that case, we believed that the patient had a bronchopleural fistula. However, in retrospect, it is more likely that hundreds of secondary and tertiary bronchioles were cut, causing a clinical picture similar to that seen with a bronchopleural fistula. In our case, considerable frothing was seen, unlike cases of bronchopleural fistulas.

Recommendation

When a bronchopleural fistula is suspected, a double-lumen tube may prove to be invaluable.

References

1. Brodsky JB. Thoracic anesthesia, Problems in anesthesia. Philadelphia: Lippincott; 1990.
2. Berry F. Anesthetic management of difficult and routine pediatric patients. New York: Churchill Livingstone; 1986. p. 167.
3. Naicker S, Brock-Utne JG, Aitchison J. Major thoracic incisional injury: ventilatory management. Anesth Analg. 1989;68:702.

Chapter 23
Case 23: Airway Leak in a Prone Patient

A 16-year-old boy (200 lb) is scheduled to donate his bone marrow under general anesthesia. The history of the donor is unremarkable except for his obesity. The patient has had no previous anesthesia/surgery, and his family history is negative for anesthesia-related complications. The patient is taking no medication and has no drug allergies. He is classified as an American Society of Anesthesiologists physical status II (ASA 2) with a class 2 airway. A 20-gauge intravenous (IV) line is placed in his left hand, and midazolam (2 mg) is given by IV in the preoperative holding area with good effect. In the operating room, after standard monitoring is placed (pulse oximetry, Dinamap, and a five-lead electrocardiogram [ECG]), he is anesthetized in a routine manner using fentanyl, thiopental, and vecuronium. Mask ventilation is found to be more difficult than was anticipated. However, when one person applies jaw thrust and another ventilates the lungs with the collapsible bag, the chest is seen to rise and the capnograph shows end-tidal CO_2. Seven minutes after the vecuronium is administered, on the third attempt, the endotracheal intubation is successful. After the airway is secured, the patient is turned prone for the surgery. Mechanical ventilation is instituted but an air hissing sound is heard stemming from the mouth. You check the pilot tubing, which seems in order. You put more air into the pilot tubing balloon, but the air leak does not go away. On auscultation, there is bilateral equal air entry. The patient's vital signs remain stable with the oxygen saturation at 100 %. The peak airway pressure is 36 cm H_2O. The air leak can still be heard 5 min after the patient is turned prone and does not seem to diminish. The leak is heard only on inspiration and not on expiration.

Questions

Will you ignore it (after all the vital signs are stable), or will you turn the patient supine and reintubate with another endotracheal tube (ETT)? Or, what will you do?

J.G. Brock-Utne, *Near Misses in Pediatric Anesthesia*,   69
DOI 10.1007/978-1-4614-7040-3_23, © Springer Science+Business Media New York 2013

Solution

You pass an orogastric tube and suck out the air that has been introduced during mask ventilation. The air leak immediately disappears. The case proceeds uneventfully, and the patient is discharged later that day.

Discussion

Gastric distension during mask ventilation is common. This is especially true for prolonged and difficult ventilation. As long as the vital signs are stable, it is worthwhile to pass an orogastric tube before considering turning the patient supine.

Recommendation

When air may have been introduced into the stomach during mask ventilation, an orogastric tube to vent the air is recommended. Even if the patient is not turned prone, decompressing the stomach may help decrease the incidence of postoperative nausea and vomiting.

Chapter 24
Case 24: Difficulty in Extubation

A 14-year-old boy (120 lb) is scheduled for an emergency appendectomy. His history is unremarkable. The patient has no previous anesthesia/surgery, and his family history is negative for anesthesia-related complications. The patient is taking no medication and is classified as an American Society of Anesthesiologists physical status I (ASA 1). General anesthesia is induced with a rapid-sequence technique including thiopental and succinylcholine after all necessary monitoring equipment is placed on the child (electrocardiogram [ECG], pulse oximeter, noninvasive blood pressure [BP], and precordial stethoscope). After the child is asleep, the trachea is intubated with a cuffed 5-mm internal diameter (i.d.) endotracheal tube (ETT). Breath sounds are equal bilaterally, and the ETT is securely taped. Anesthesia is maintained with isoflurane and nitrous oxide in oxygen, meperidine, and vecuronium. The operation proceeds uneventfully, and at the end of the surgery the neuromuscular blockade is reversed. Spontaneous respiration returns, but the patient is unable to follow commands. He is therefore transported to the postanesthesia care unit (PACU) recovery room with the ETT still in place.

Shortly after arriving in the PACU, the patient becomes alert. He attempts to remove the ETT from the trachea. In your attempt to rapidly deflate the ETT cuff, the pilot balloon and the valve assembly are pulled off the pilot tube. In so doing, the pilot tube is stretched, occluding the stump of the tube that is still attached to the inflated cuff. The cuff is therefore still inflated and, despite several attempts, the ETT cannot be removed.

Questions

What will you do initially? How will you remove the ETT atraumatically?

J.G. Brock-Utne, *Near Misses in Pediatric Anesthesia*,
DOI 10.1007/978-1-4614-7040-3_24, © Springer Science+Business Media New York 2013

Solution

The patient must be verbally reassured and encouraged to breathe easily through the ETT. Sedation may be necessary.

You have the following options:

1. Deflate the cuff with a syringe and needle inserted past the occlusion in the stump of the pilot tube.
2. Puncture the cuff with a needle either during direct observation using a laryngoscope or indirectly through the cricothyroid membrane.
3. Cut the pilot tube proximal to the obstruction, thereby letting the air out.

Discussion

This case is similar to a previous report [1]. Other causes of difficult extubation include inadvertently having the ETT wired to facial bones [2], sutured to the pulmonary artery [3], transfixed by a screw [4], stuck to the tracheal mucosa because of absence of lubricant [5], wrapped up in the nasogastric tube [6], and fixed below the cords by folds in the deflated cuff [7, 8]. Another case of difficult extubation involved an ETT with a self-inflating cuff that became trapped when the cuff tube broke off, preventing deflation [9].

Recommendation

The practice of pulling off the pilot balloon and valve assembly to deflate the tracheal cuff should be strongly discouraged. Besides the complication recorded here, there is the situation in which an emergency reintubation of a recently extubated patient is needed. If no other ETT is available, then the ETT, which is just removed from the patient and intact, can be used again.

References

1. Brock-Utne JG, Jaffe RA, Robins B, Ratner E. Difficulty in extubation. Anaesthesia. 1992;47:229–30.
2. Lee C, Schwartz S, Mok MS. Difficult extubation due to transfixation of a nasotracheal tube by a Kirschner wire. Anesthesiology. 1977;46:427.
3. Dryden GE. Circulatory collapse after pneumonectomy (an unusual complication from the use of a Carlens catheter). Anesth Analg. 1997;56:451–2.
4. Lang S, Johnson DH, Lanigan DT, Hang H. Difficult tracheal extubation. Can J Anaesth. 1989;36:340–2.

5. Debain JJ, Le Brigand H, Binet JP, Pottemain M, Freyss G, Bonhomme F. Quelques incidents et accidents de l'intubation trachéale prolongée: étude des résultats d'ensemble dans un service de chirurgie cardio-pulmonaire et dans un service de réanimation médicale (Some difficulties and accidents of prolonged tracheal intubation: study of combined results in a cardiopulmonary department and in a medical resuscitation department). Ann Otolaryngol Chir Cervicofac. 1968;85:379–86.
6. Fagraes L. Difficult extubation following nasotracheal intubation. Anesthesiology. 1978;49: 43–4.
7. Ng TY, Datta TD. Difficult extubation of an endotracheal tube cuff. Anesth Analg. 1976;55: 876–7.
8. Mishra P, Scott DL. Difficulty at extubation of the trachea. Anaesthesia. 1983;38:811.
9. Tavakoli M, Corssen G. An unusual case of difficult extubation. Anesthesiology. 1976; 45:552–3.

Chapter 25
Case 25: Tonsillectomy

Today the pharmacy tells you that there is no sevoflurane available. Fortunately, the bioengineer finds a halothane vaporizer and after checking the anesthesia machine you agree to proceed.

The first case of the day is a 2-year-old boy who presents for tonsillectomy. His medical history is negative with the exception of numerous bouts of tonsillitis. A hernia repair under general anesthesia at the age of 1 year was uneventful. He is classified American Society of Anesthesiologists physical status I (ASA 1). An oral midazolam premedication is given with good effect. His vital signs in the operating room show a heart rate of 90 beats per minute (bpm), regular sinus rhythm, blood pressure (BP) of 110/50, and oxygen saturation of 100 %. A mask induction, as per patient's request, is commenced with 100 % oxygen in halothane up to 4 %. Within 2–3 min, the patient is asleep with normal vital signs. Mask ventilation with halothane 2 % commences and an intravenous (IV) line is inserted. Before any drugs are given, there is a sudden loss of oximetry pulseform and the alarm goes off. Adequate chest exertion is seen with manual ventilation. The electrocardiogram (ECG) shows a regular sinus heart rate of 76 bpm. You feel for pulses superficial temporal, carotid, and femoral artery. But there is none. The ECG still shows 76 bpm.

Questions

Are you concerned? If so, what will you do?

J.G. Brock-Utne, *Near Misses in Pediatric Anesthesia*,
DOI 10.1007/978-1-4614-7040-3_25, © Springer Science+Business Media New York 2013

Solution

1. Turn the halothane off.
2. Commence cardiopulmonary resuscitation with 100 % oxygen via mask airway.
3. Call for a defibrillator.
4. Perform endotracheal intubation.

After these measures, the femoral pulse reappeared, and the oxygen saturation improved to 100 % with rebound hypertension. Despite the fact that you could feel the pulse to be over 120 bpm, the ECG still showed a regular sinus heart rate of 76 bpm. The oximeter also showed a pulse of 126 bpm. A decision to proceed with the operation was made after a new ECG machine was attached to the patient. This machine now showed the pulse to be also 126 bpm. No further problems arose during the operation, and the patient was awakened and seen to be neurologically intact. A benign course in the hospital followed, and the patient was discharged the next day.

Discussion

One can only speculate as to what happened, but it is most likely that an overdose of halothane (without preoperative atropine) led to a severe, rapid-onset bradycardia and arrhythmia. On inspection of the ECG machine, it was noted to be a demonstration model on loan to the hospital. The monitor was configured such that if no pulse was detected, it automatically went into a demonstration mode (e.g., sinus rhythm of 76 bpm). If the physical examination had not been done, or delayed, the outcome of this case would have been very different.

Recommendation

When in doubt, examine your patient. If you find no pulses, then there are no pulses despite an ECG that tells you otherwise.

Chapter 26
Case 26: An Unusual Cause of a Serious Cardiac Arrhythmia

A 17-year-old boy (American Society of Anesthesiologists physical status II [ASA 2]) with a diagnosis of a chronic pain syndrome involving his right chest as a result of a motorbike accident is scheduled for a dorsal root entry zone (DREZ) lesion placement at right T10, T11, and T12 with dermatomal evoked potential monitoring. The patient's history includes several back surgical procedures. In the preoperative area, midazolam, 4 mg intravenous (IV), is given for sedation. Monitors are placed on the patient in the operating room, and anesthesia is induced using thiopental, fentanyl, and vecuronium. After the airway is secured, the patient is turned prone onto a Wilson frame, and all pressure points are padded. Anesthesia is maintained with isoflurane, nitrous oxide, vecuronium, and meperidine. Anesthesia monitors consist of noninvasive blood pressure (BP), electrocardiogram (ECG), pulse oximetry, esophageal stethoscope, temperature probe, oxygen analyzer, and end-tidal CO_2. The neurologist uses the Hewlett-Packard Component Monitoring System, model M10948 (Mountain View, CA). The ECG skin electrodes from 3M Health Care Red Dot, model 2238 (St. Paul, MN), are placed as follows: right arm lead (white) at the right posterior shoulder, left arm lead (black) at the left posterior shoulder, right leg lead (green) at the right midaxillary line at the sixth intercostal space, left leg lead (red) at the left midaxillary line at the eighth intercostal space, and the V_5 lead (brown) at the left midaxillary line at the fifth intercostal space. Evoked potential stimulator skin electrodes are placed at the right T8, T10, T12, and the left T10 dermatomes by the neurologist. Using a Nicolet Viking IV (Madison, WI), the neurologist will monitor evoked potentials, after dermatomal electrical stimulation, to help evaluate the efficacy of the placement of the DREZ lesions by the surgeons.

Forty minutes after surgery begins, ECG changes consistent with supraventricular tachycardia (282 beats per minute [bpm]) are observed (Fig. 26.1); however, his pulse by palpation, esophageal stethoscope, and pulse oximeter is 84 bpm and regular. Furthermore, the patient's oxygen saturation is 100 %, and his BP is unchanged at 120/80. A search for possible causes is undertaken, but within 60 s the ECG returns to normal sinus rhythm with a rate of 84 bpm (Fig. 26.2). His vital signs continue to remain stable, but a few minutes later the phenomenon reappears and, again, lasts less than 1 min. No surgery is being done nor is the electrocautery being used.

J.G. Brock-Utne, *Near Misses in Pediatric Anesthesia*, 77
DOI 10.1007/978-1-4614-7040-3_26, © Springer Science+Business Media New York 2013

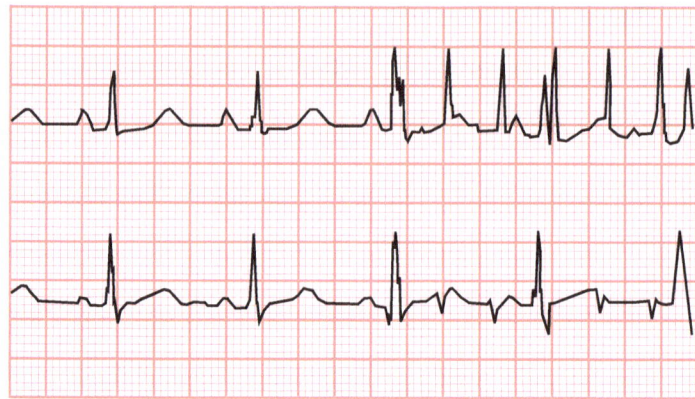

Fig. 26.1 Electrocardiographic changes observed in lead II (*upper trace*). Lead V$_5$ is shown in *lower trace*. Reproduced with permission from Diachun CAB, Brock-Utne JG, Lopez JR, Ceranski J. Evoked potential monitoring and EKG: a case of a serious "cardiac arrhythmia". Anesthesiology. 1998;89;1270–2

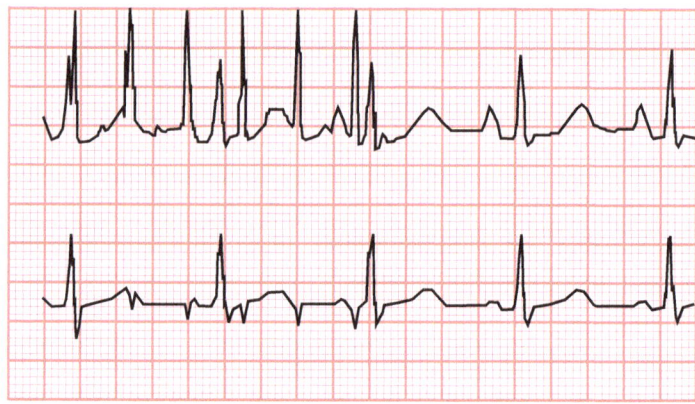

Fig. 26.2 Electrocardiographic trace with lead II (*upper trace*) shows return to normal sinus rhythm. Lead V$_5$ is shown in *lower trace*. Reproduced with permission from Diachun CAB, Brock-Utne JG, Lopez JR, Ceranski J. Evoked potential monitoring and EKG: a case of a serious "cardiac arrhythmia". Anesthesiology. 1998;89;1270–2

You check the blood gas and electrolyte levels, which are all within normal limits, but the ECG changes consistent with supraventricular tachycardia reoccur and disappear at intervals, with all other parameters remaining normal.

Questions

What will you do? Ignore it or treat it?

Solution

The best thing to do is ask the neurologist who is monitoring the evoked potentials to stimulate the dermatomes. Most likely, you will see a supraventricular tachycardia–like ECG (see Fig. 26.1). This has been reported in an adult patient [1]. In that case, we believed that the positioning of our ECG electrodes in close proximity to the evoked potential–stimulating electrodes caused the nearly equal amplitude of the evoked potential deflections to that of our QRS complex in our inferior leads.

Discussion

During ECG recording, the skin electrodes detect voltage changes that are displayed graphically. These voltage changes reflect the electrical current produced during cardiac depolarization and repolarization. Interference patterns are often observed on ECG monitors, even with signal filtering [2]. Most commonly, interference is observed with electrocautery use [2]. However, Kimberly et al. [3] and Sliwa and Marinko [4] have described interference on ECGs from transcutaneous nerve stimulators (TENS) with electrodes placed parasternally and at the lower thoracic and lumbar regions.

Somatosensory evoked potentials are produced by electrical stimulation of a selected peripheral nerve at an intensity sufficient to cause a twitch of the muscles supplied by that nerve. Recording electrodes placed over the peripheral nerve, lumbar spine, brachial plexus, cervical spine, and scalp detect the electrical potentials that traverse the sensory neural tracts from the periphery to the central nervous system. Changes in the amplitude or latency of these potentials may indicate damage to the neural tracts. During previous cases in which evoked potential monitoring has been used, we have often observed interference patterns represented by small sharp deflections on the ECG trace. In those instances, the stimulating electrodes were placed at the wrists, in contrast to this case, in which the electrodes were placed on the patient's torso. A similar electrical interference pattern was reported by Sliwa and Marinko with TENS electrode stimulation [4]. The most frequent interference pattern we have observed during past evoked potential monitoring is shown in the lateral lead V_5 trace (see Figs. 26.1 and 26.2). This more usual interference pattern can easily be misinterpreted as pacemaker spikes. In fact, Sliwa and Marinko [4] report that this type of interference was interpreted by a reading cardiologist as a malfunctioning pacemaker.

Recommendation

This case cautions the reader that evoked potential monitoring can lead to false signals of cardiac arrhythmias that should be confirmed as interference. The case illustrates the all-important dogma: "Always treat the patient and *not* the monitors."

It is of great importance not to overreact to an "abnormal" monitoring parameter. When in doubt, examine the patient and then review all other monitors to confirm possible disaster. Serious problems can occur when one elects to treat a nonexistent arrhythmia.

References

1. Diachun CAB, Brock-Utne JG, Lopes JR, Ceranski J. Evoked potential monitoring and EKG: a case of a serious "cardiac arrhythmia". Anesthesiology. 1998;89:1270–2.
2. Barash PG, Cullen BE, Stoelting RK. Clinical anesthesia. 2nd ed. Philadelphia: Lippincott; 1992. pp. 760–1, 771–5, 1067–8.
3. Kimberly APS, Soni N, Williams TR. Transcutaneous nerve stimulation and the electrocardiograph. Anaesth Intensive Care. 1987;15:358–9.
4. Sliwa JA, Marinko MS. Transcutaneous electrical nerve stimulator-induced electrocardiogram artifact: a brief report. Am J Phys Med Rehabil. 1996;75:307–9.

Chapter 27
Case 27: A Patient with Supraglottic Mass

A 2-year-old child is scheduled for pharyngoscopy and biopsy for a pharyngeal mass. The child is breathless but has no stridor. The mouth opening is adequate, with a good view of the uvula. The chest X-ray is normal, and the lateral X-ray of the soft tissues of the neck shows a large supraglottic soft-tissue mass. This mass projects from the posterior pharyngeal wall into the larynx, which is narrowed by approximately 70 %.

The patient is taken to the operating theater, where an intravenous (IV) line and standard monitoring are started. In the event of an airway crisis, an emergency tracheostomy set is available. Inhalation induction with sevoflurane and oxygen is commenced. Induction of general anesthesia is well tolerated. Airway obstruction occurs suddenly as muscle tone is lost. Repositioning of the jaw and head does not improve the obstruction, nor does the introduction of an oral airway, and a laryngeal mask airway (LMA) cannot be passed. The patient's oxygen saturation continues to fall, sevoflurane induction is stopped, and the child is awakened from the general anesthetic.

A tracheostomy under regional block with sedation is not considered an option because sedation could cause severe respiratory depression. The pediatric fiber-optic laryngoscope is found to be nonfunctioning.

Question

What will you do now?

J.G. Brock-Utne, *Near Misses in Pediatric Anesthesia*,
DOI 10.1007/978-1-4614-7040-3_27, © Springer Science+Business Media New York 2013

Solution

Inhalation induction with sevoflurane and oxygen was again performed. When the muscle tone was lost, airway obstruction occurred again. The skin over the entire cartilage was grabbed and gently lifted upward. The obstruction was immediately relieved. Spontaneous ventilation resumed, and anesthesia was deepened further. When the skin over the laryngeal cartilage was released, obstruction reoccurred. The skin was again lifted up, and the airway became patent. When anesthesia depth was considered adequate, laryngoscopy was performed and the postsupra-glottic mass was seen overlying the glottis. A 3.5-mm internal diameter (i.d.) uncuffed tracheal tube was passed easily. Oxygen desaturation did not occur, and no muscle relaxation was administered. The tumor was biopsied and debulked. After return of consciousness, extubation was performed with the child in the right lateral position.

Recommendation

This simple technique should be tried when airway obstruction occurs during inhalation induction in a patient with a supraglottic tumor.

Chapter 28
Case 28: Pressurized Intravenous Hetastarch

A 2-year-old child is taken to the operating room for an emergency laparotomy. Four hours earlier, the child had a kidney tumor removed, uneventfully, under general anesthesia. On examination, the child is pale, cold, and clammy, with a heart rate of 150 beats per minute (bpm) and a systolic blood pressure (BP) of 60 mmHg. The intravenous (IV) line in his left arm is seen to work adequately. Air is noted in the half-filled 6 % Hetastarch bag (Abbott Laboratories, North Chicago, IL). The child is anesthetized with ketamine, suxamethonium, and cricoid pressure. An endotracheal tube (ETT) is inserted atraumatically, and breath sounds are equal bilaterally. Anesthesia is maintained with air in oxygen 50/50, fentanyl, and isoflurane. After the abdomen is opened, the BP falls precipitously and the Hespan bag is pressurized. Blood that was requested has not arrived. Suddenly the end-tidal CO_2 falls from 46 to 20 mmHg. The pulse is 140 and the BP is 50/30. The oxygen saturation (99 %) remains unchanged.

Questions

Are you concerned? If so, what will you do?

J.G. Brock-Utne, *Near Misses in Pediatric Anesthesia*,
DOI 10.1007/978-1-4614-7040-3_28, © Springer Science+Business Media New York 2013

Solution

You notice air in the IV tubing and stop the Hetastarch infusion. The air seen in the Hetastarch bag preoperatively was overlooked and forgotten at the time of induction and subsequent pressurization of the bag [1]. Normally, IV bags have no air, only fluid. If the IV bags are punctured with a giving set more than once, there is a high risk of getting air into the bag. In this case, the air volume infused was considered small (no more than 40 ml) and the end-tidal CO_2 gradually recovered over a period of minutes.

Discussion

The lethal dose of intravascular air in humans is unknown, but accidental injections of between 100 and 300 ml have been known to be fatal. The cause of death from massive air embolus is circulatory obstruction with cardiovascular collapse resulting from air trapped in the right ventricular outflow tract.

I have seen a patient die from air embolism caused by air infused from a 500-ml glass blood bottle (an unknown amount of air, but thought to be at least 500 ml). Be aware that in many parts of the world, human blood is still provided in glass bottles. Blood in glass bottles can only be forced out rapidly into the patient by pressurizing the inside of the bottle with air. If a watchful eye is not kept on the blood levels in the giving set, air can easily be forced into the patient's circulation. Failure to be observant in these cases can lead to large quantities of air being forced into the patient—quantities sufficient to cause death.

Recommendation

All air must be expelled from all plastic IV bottles before they are used, especially if the bag is pressurized. If all the air cannot be removed, then throw away the IV bag. This is especially true in pediatrics.

Reference

1. Baldwin AM, Roberts JG. Air embolism following infusion of Haemaccel. Anaesth Intensive Care. 1991;19:130–1.

Chapter 29
Case 29: Intraoperative Hypotension

A 5-year-old boy (12 kg) with a 36-h history of nausea and vomiting is admitted to the hospital. The child has a history of hydrocephalus and seizure disorder. A ventriculoperitoneal shunt, placed uneventfully under general anesthesia several years before, is seen to be working adequately. His medication consists of carbamazepine, 20 mg/kg per day. The patient has no history of drug allergy, nor is there any adverse family history of anesthetic complications. On examination, the child is listless, with other clinical signs of hypovolemia (skin turgor, mucous membranes, peripheral shut down). A chest X-ray shows bowel in the left hemithorax, and a presumptive diagnosis of a hernia of Morgagni is made. A pediatric surgeon is called. The child is rehydrated over a 2-h period and the blood electrolytes are normal. A rapid-sequence induction/intubation is performed without any difficulty (ketamine, 20 mg, and rocuronium, 20 mg) at 3:00 AM. Anesthesia is maintained with oxygen in air and isoflurane 0.3–0.5 %. A thoracic epidural catheter is placed 15 min later, and 9 ml of 0.25 % bupivacaine with 0.2 mg hydromorphone (Dilaudid) is injected. At 3:30 AM, cefazolin (Kefzol), 500 mg intravenous (IV), is administered, and at 4:15 AM, the surgeons have full exposure of the hernia through a laparotomy incision. At 4:20 AM, the blood pressure (BP) drops precipitously, with hardly a change in heart rate. Peak inspired pressure and tidal volume are not changed. The SPO_2 is 100 % on 100 % FIO_2, and his temperature is normal. Ephedrine, 2 mg, has no effect, and the BP drops to 50 mmHg. Epinephrine, 5–20 μ(mu)g, is used to maintain the BP. The heart rate drops from 110 to 80. You consider the following causes of this intraoperative hypotension: overdose of bupivacaine and/or of inhalation anesthetic and allergic reactions to muscle relaxants and/or antibiotics.

Questions

Are there any other causes you would consider? If so, what will you do?

J.G. Brock-Utne, *Near Misses in Pediatric Anesthesia*,
DOI 10.1007/978-1-4614-7040-3_29, © Springer Science+Business Media New York 2013

Solution

Consider latex allergy. If possible, attempt to see if the patient has any generalized rash or flushing of the skin. Although not specific for latex allergy, it does point to the fact that you most likely have a patient with serious intraoperative anaphylaxis. In this case, the patient was severely flushed. The suggested management of a potential latex allergy is as follows:

1. Remove any latex materials. The surgeon must change gloves.
2. Ventilate with 100 % oxygen.
3. Consider aborting procedure.
4. Administer non-sugar-containing fluid (5–10 ml/kg IV bolus followed by 10–20 ml/kg per hour).
5. Administer epinephrine, 2–6 µg/kg IV bolus, for hypotension, then 0.1–0.5 µg/kg in 250 ml normal saline IV infusion; titrate to effect for hypotension or bronchospasms.
6. Take several samples of blood for tryptase measurements [1], IgE antibodies, and complement C3 and C4.

Discussion

Latex is the milky sap that comes from a tree in the Amazon River region and is used in the manufacture of natural rubber products. Latex products include catheters and surgical gloves. Even so-called hypoallergenic gloves have small quantities of latex in them.

In a study of 18 cases of intraoperative anaphylaxis attributed to latex, the earliest time of onset occurred 40 min after induction of anesthesia. Many reactions occurred much later [2]. In this case, it took 75 min. In contrast, 80 % of most other anesthetic drug-induced anaphylactic reactions occurred at or shortly after induction of a general anesthesia, within a few minutes of administration of the offending drug [3, 4].

An adverse reaction to latex requires a period of time before a systemic reaction is seen, because the responsible allergenic protein must be eluted from the rubber gloves and absorbed into the circulation in sufficient amounts before a systemic reaction is seen. Slater et al. [5] found that 34 % of children with spina bifida had serum antibodies specific for latex rubber protein. The case of contact urticaria due to latex rubber was first reported in 1979 [6], and intraoperative anaphylaxis associated with latex sensitivity was first reported in 1984 [7].

A patient who has previously suffered systemic reaction should not be given provocation tests [8]. Skin prick testing is often used when one suspects a latex allergy.

Braude et al. [9] identified a specific group of pediatric patients at risk for latex anaphylaxis, including patients with either spina bifida or congenital urologic abnormalities who have been exposed to latex products on an intermittent basis.

Recommendation

Information that patients are latex sensitive or suspected of having a latex sensitivity (as indicated if the child is allergic to balloons) should always be taken very seriously. A pretreatment regimen is not advisable, as one study has shown it is not effective [2].

References

1. Blanco I, Cardenas E, Aguilera L, Camino E, Arizaga A, Telletxea S. Serum tryptase measurement in diagnosis of intraoperative anaphylaxis caused by hydatid cyst. Anaesth Intensive Care. 1996;24:489–91.
2. Gold M, Swartz JS, Braude BM, Dolovich J, Shandling B, Gilmour RF. Intraoperative anaphylaxis: an association with latex sensitivity. J Allergy Clin Immunol. 1991;87:662–6.
3. Moscicki RA, Sockin SM, Corsello BF, Ostro MG, Bloch KJ. Anaphylaxis during induction of general anesthesia: subsequent evaluation and management. J Allergy Clin Immunol. 1990;86: 325–31.
4. Fisher MM, More DG. The epidemiology and clinical features of anaphylactic reaction in anaesthesia. Anaesth Intensive Care. 1981;9:226–34.
5. Slater JE, Mostello LA, Shaer C. Rubber-specific IgE in children with spina bifida. J Urol. 1991;146:578–9.
6. Nutter AF. Contact urticaria to rubber. Br J Dermatol. 1979;101:597–8.
7. Sethna NF, Sockin SM, Holzman RS, Slater JE. Latex anaphylaxis in a child with a history of multiple anesthetic drug allergies. Anesthesiology. 1992;77:372–5.
8. Turjarimaa K, Reunala T, Rasanen L. Comparison of diagnostic methods in latex surgical glove contact urticaria. Contact Dermatitis. 1988;19:241–7.
9. Swartz JS, Gold M, Braude BM, Dolovich J, Gilmour RF, Shandling B. Intraoperative anaphylaxis to latex: an identifiable population at risk. Can J Anaesth. 1990;37(4 Pt 2):S131.

Chapter 30
Case 30: Hematuria

A 17-year-old girl (120 lb) presents with hematuria and is scheduled for a cystostomy. Her history is unremarkable except for interstitial cystitis. The patient has had numerous anesthesia/surgery procedures for her complaints. The family history is negative for anesthesia-related complications. The patient is taking no medication and is classified as an American Society of Anesthesiologists physical status I (ASA 1). The patient requests an epidural anesthetic, and as there are no contraindications, an epidural is placed in L3–L4 interspace. Lidocaine 2 % (15 ml) produces a good block, and the operation proceeds uneventfully. Thirty-five minutes after the start of the surgery, the patient complains that she is feeling unwell. You have given no drugs for the last 50 min. You note that the electrocardiogram (ECG) shows a sudden onset of ventricular tachycardia and the Dynamap alarms, indicating no blood pressure (BP). The oxygen saturation has dropped from 100 % to 76 %. The patient is now unconscious and, although you do not know what happened, you quickly place a face mask with 100 % oxygen and assist her respiration. The carotid pulse is present but very weak. The Dynamap still indicates no BP. The saturation has increased to 86 %. You call for a defibrillator and proceed to deliver a shock at 100 J. There is a rapid return to sinus tachycardia, and the BP returns to normal as does oxygen saturation. The patient complains of pain in the chest and inquires as to what happened. You are at a loss to explain the cause. The epidural lidocaine that you gave 35 min ago is highly unlikely to be the cause.

Question

What do you think the possible cause is for this sudden turn of events?

J.G. Brock-Utne, *Near Misses in Pediatric Anesthesia*,
DOI 10.1007/978-1-4614-7040-3_30, © Springer Science+Business Media New York 2013

Solution

In this case, the surgeon was asked if he had done anything. After some time and several prompting questions, the surgeon admitted that he had injected epinephrine (1,000 μ[mu]g) into the bladder wall. This he had done for hemostasis.

Discussion

When unexplained problems arise intraoperatively, it is important that you make certain that you have not done anything that can be the cause of the problem. Having exhausted all of your causes, it is time to ask the surgeon.

The surgeon and the anesthesiologist should always keep each other informed during the intraoperative period as to problems or concerns. If the surgeon had told the anesthesiologist that the patient had excessive bleeding and was considering using epinephrine, then this problem could have been avoided. Needless to say, this patient will always remember that she had a shock during surgery.

Recommendation

Surgeons should always inform the anesthesiologist about the drug concentration and amount they are giving intraoperatively.

Chapter 31
Case 31: Congenital Complete Heart Block

A 10-year-old boy (25 kg) with signs and symptoms of acute appendicitis is admitted to the hospital. The child has a history of congenital complete heart block (CCHB). The heart condition, however, does not interfere with the child's activity. There is no history of cardiac failure or syncope. The patient has no history of drug allergy or previous general anesthesia, nor any adverse family history of anesthetic complications. On examination, the child is found to be otherwise healthy. Heart rate is 50 beats per minute (bpm). A low-grade systolic murmur is heard at the apex. Blood pressure (BP) is 100/60 mmHg, and the chest is clear. The electrocardiogram (ECG) shows a complete heart block. The chest X-ray is normal. You request a transvenous pacemaker, but none is available. Transferring the patient to another hospital is not an option because it is more than 4 h away.

Question

How will you proceed?

J.G. Brock-Utne, *Near Misses in Pediatric Anesthesia*, 91
DOI 10.1007/978-1-4614-7040-3_31, © Springer Science+Business Media New York 2013

Solution

The following drugs and equipment should be readily available: atropine and iso-proterenol to treat bradycardia, and lidocaine and a direct current (DC) defibrillator in case of ventricular arrhythmia. Remember that many of the new DC defibrillators have the ability to act as transcutaneous external pacemakers. These are very useful in cases of extreme bradycardia or cardiac standstill. No preoperative orogastric tube should be used because it can cause bradycardia.

A previous case report [1] has recommended the following general anesthesia regimen with some modifications: (1) atropine and meperidine given preoperatively, (2) a rapid-sequence induction/intubation with ketamine and rocuronium, and (3) anesthesia maintained with oxygen in nitrous oxide and isoflurane.

In the aforementioned case report, the pulse was kept at 100 bpm. At the end of the procedure, the neuromuscular block was reversed with atropine (1.0 mg), followed a minute later by neostigmine (2 mg). The patient had an uneventful recovery with a pulse rate remaining between 60 and 70 bpm, with complete atrioventricular dissociation persisting throughout his hospital stay.

Discussion

Uncomplicated forms of CCHB are compatible with completely normal development. Some patients exhibit acceleration of a junctional pacemaker, producing a near-normal heart rate with exercise [2]. This is presumed to be the case reported here. Usually, however, CCHB may be associated with serious congenital cardiac defects like a single ventricle, ventricular septal defects, or transposition of the great vessels [3]. The majority of children with CCHB can be managed successfully with adequate vagolysis and avoidance of drugs that have negative chronotropic effects [4]. Steward and Izukawa have recommended that all patients with CCHB have transvenous pacemakers inserted before induction of general anesthesia [5]; however, transvenous pacemakers are not without problems. Diza and Friesen recommend that it may be more logical to use transvenous pacemakers if there is a history of exercise intolerance, congestive cardiac failure, and a QRS interval of more than 0.1 s. Whatever the plan adopted, one must always have isoproterenol and preferably a transcutaneous external pacemaker readily available. How important drugs like atropine, meperidine, and isoflurane are in producing tachycardia during anesthesia is speculative.

Recommendation

In patients with CCHB who are to undergo general anesthesia, a detailed history and examination are mandatory. Depending on the above finding, a general anesthesia plan that may include a transvenous pacemaker should be made. In any case, isoproterenol intravenous (IV) drip and a transcutaneous external pacemaker/defibrillator must be readily available.

References

1. Duffy BL. Congenital complete heart block. General anaesthesia for appendectomy in an adolescent (case report). Anaesthesia. 1981;36:956–7.
2. Sobel BE, Braunwald E. Cardiac dysrhythmias. In: Isselbacher KJ, Adams RD, Braunwald E, et al., editors. Harrison's principles of internal medicine. 9th ed. New York: McGraw-Hill; 1980;1044–63.
3. Hurst JW. Cardiac arrhythmias and conduction disturbances. In: Hurst JW, editor. The heart. 3rd ed. New York: McGraw-Hill; 1974;495–569.
4. Diaz JH, Friesen RH. Anesthetic management of congenital complete heart block in childhood. Anesth Analg. 1979;58:334–6.
5. Steward DJ, Izukawa T. Congenital complete heart block. Anesth Analg. 1980;59:81.

Chapter 32
Case 32: Neonatal Respiratory Distress

A premature (32 weeks' gestation), 2.1-kg boy is admitted to the pediatric intensive care unit (ICU) shortly after birth. He has intercostal and substernal recession. Cyanosis is evident even with FIO_2 of 0.5. No congenital abnormalities are seen. Auscultation of the chest confirms the presence of bilateral air entry with widespread crepitations. Chest X-ray shows that most of the lungs are not aerated. A diagnosis of respiratory failure (hyaline membrane disease associated with prematurity) is made. Despite treatment, the infant does not improve and the condition becomes grave, with an arterial pH of 7.0, PaO_2 of 55 mmHg, and a $PaCO_2$ of 90 mmHg. You intubate the infant's trachea with a 3-mm tube and provide intermittent positive pressure of the lungs. The FIO_2 is 0.6, the rate is 30 per minute, and a 3-cm positive end-expiratory pressure is provided. There is dramatic improvement in the infant's condition within 1–2 h. A new chest X-ray also shows improvement. You note that there seems to be evidence of bifid spines in the lower cervical and upper thoracic regions.

Question

Would you investigate the bifid spines further and, if so, what will you do?

Solution

A lateral chest X-ray should be taken. In this case, the esophagus and trachea were seen to be displaced anterior from the vertebral column. These findings, together with the bifid spines, make the diagnosis of a large neuroenteric cyst very likely. In a previous case report [1], a large cyst was removed. The cyst appeared to originate from the upper thoracic vertebrae, where it was narrow, and from there expanded to fill the space posterior to the mediastinum. In that case, the recovery was uneventful, and the child was discharged on day 10.

Discussion

The rapid improvement after intermittent positive pressure ventilation made the diagnosis of hyaline membrane disease unlikely. Hence, this case illustrates the importance of reviewing the information on which the first diagnosis was based. Neonatal distress due to mediastinal tumors is extremely uncommon [2] and neuro-enteric cysts account for only 3 % of all mediastinal tumors [3]. Neuroenteric cysts are considered to originate from a split notochord [4] and are associated with spinal abnormalities [3, 5]. The diagnosis of these cysts is usually made on the basis of the presence of a fluid-filled cyst, abnormal vertebrae, and a forward displacement of the mediastinum. Air bronchogram, a feature of hyaline membrane disease, does not occur.

Recommendation

When a dramatic, unexpected clinical improvement occurs, a review of the diagnosis is imperative. In a case such as this, always remember to look at the bony structures, even in a chest X-ray.

References

1. Cahill JF. An unusual cause of neonatal respiratory distress. Anaesthesia. 1981;36:790–4.
2. Seibert JJ, Marvin WJ, Rose EF, Schienken RM. Mediastinal teratoma: a rare cause of severe respiratory distress in the newborn. J Paediatr Surg. 1976;11:253–5.
3. Kirwan WO, Walbaum PR, McCormac RJM. Cystic intrathoracic derivatives of the foregut and their complications. Thorax. 1973;28:424–8.
4. Caffey J. Paediatric X-ray diagnosis, vol. 1. 6th ed. London: Lloyd-Luke; 1972;642–4.
5. Fallon M, Gordon ARG, Ledrum AC. Mediastinal cysts of fore-gut origin associated with vertebral abnormalities. Br J Surg. 1954;41:520–33.

Chapter 33
Case 33: Respiratory Distress in the Intensive Care Unit

A 16-year-old boy is admitted to the intensive care unit (ICU) after a motor vehicle accident. He has suffered a concussion and contusion of the left lung. He is receiving assisted ventilation via an endotracheal tube (ETT). In the ICU, a hemopneumothorax is diagnosed and a left chest tube is placed. An extensive tracheobronchial toilet is performed, and 200 ml of bloodstained fluid is aspirated. The patient is very restless and is sedated with midazolam, vecuronium, and morphine. After 3 days, an attempt is made to wean him from the ventilator. Unfortunately, he bites on the ETT so that the ETT obstructs. A bite block is inserted, but the patient spits it out. A Fergusson mouth gag is used with good effect as the jaws are kept apart. Further reduction in sedation is now possible; however, a few hours later he suddenly becomes very restless and manages to extubate the ETT himself. The mouth gag is removed. Initially, his respiration is adequate. Within a few hours, however, there is clinical evidence of collapse of the left lung. Chest X-ray shows hyperinflation of the right lung and collapse of the left lung with a possible foreign body lodged in the left main bronchus. At bronchoscopy, a foreign body is removed.

Question

What is the foreign object and what could have been done to prevent this mishap?

Solution

The foreign body was a rubber sleeve from one of the jaws of the mouth gag. This case is similar to a reported case (shown in Fig. 33.1) [1].

Discussion

There are a number of reports of various pieces of anesthetic equipment that have been lodged in the tracheobronchial tree with potentially dangerous ramifications [1–3]. In this case, the mouth gag was removed, but no one noticed that one of the rubber sleeves was missing. We have reported a case in which the tip of the Bullard laryngoscope was left behind, with potentially serious complications [4]. Stressed in the Bullard manuscript is the need for understanding any equipment and its limitations, and to always read the instructions before using it.

Recommendation

All items that have been in the airway should always be inspected to see if they are intact on removal. Anything left behind can have potentially serious consequences.

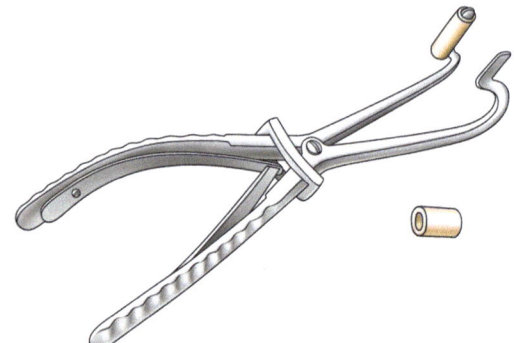

Fig. 33.1 Fergusson mouth gag. Reproduced with permission from Mulligan IP, Marshall RD. Inhalation of a foreign body. A hazard of protective rubber sleeves on the jaws of mouth gags. Anesthesia. 1981;36:800–2

References

1. Mulligan IP, Marshall RD. Inhalation of a foreign body. A hazard of protective rubber sleeves on the jaws of mouth gags. Anesthesia. 1981;36:800–2.
2. Saijo S, Tomioka S, Takasaka T, Kawamoto K. Foreign bodies in the tracheobronchial tree. A review of 110 cases. Arch Otorhinolaryngol. 1979;225:1–7.
3. Kamholz SL, Rothman NI, Underwood PS. Fiberbronchoscopie retrieval of iatrogenically introduced endobronchial foreign body. Crit Care Med. 1979;7:346–8.
4. Habibi A, Bushell E, Jaffe RA, Giffard R, Brock-Utne JG. Two tips for the Bullard intubating laryngoscope. Anesth Analg. 1998;87:1206–8.

Suggested Reading

Donnelly LF, Frush DP, Bisset GS. The multiple presentations of foreign bodies in children. Am J Roentgenol. 1998;170:471477.

Chapter 34
Case 34: The Butterfly Needle (Abbott)

A 3-year-old boy (34 lb) is scheduled for an urgent manipulation of a fractured forearm. He has just come from a birthday party and has eaten cake and other sweets within the last hour. His medical history is unremarkable. The patient has no known drug allergies, and the family history is negative for anesthesia-related problems. An intravenous (IV) (25-gauge) Butterfly needle is established in the back of the hand with the help of lidocaine/prilocaine (EMLA cream). Monitoring equipment is placed on the child (electrocardiogram [ECG], pulse oximeter, a nerve stimulator, noninvasive blood pressure [BP], and precordial stethoscope). General anesthesia is induced with propofol (35 mg) followed by succinylcholine (20 mg) using the Butterfly needle to good effect. The patient's trachea is easily intubated, and general anesthesia is initially maintained with isoflurane 1–3 % with 70 % nitrous oxide in oxygen. After 10 min, with the patient breathing spontaneously, meperidine, 10 mg, is injected again through the Butterfly needle. A few seconds later, the pulse oximeter alarms and the ECG shows a bradycardia of 40 beats per minute (bpm). You are puzzled because meperidine, being an atropine derivative, should produce a tachycardia, not a bradycardia.

Question

What is the cause of the bradycardia and what will you do?

J.G. Brock-Utne, *Near Misses in Pediatric Anesthesia*,
DOI 10.1007/978-1-4614-7040-3_34, © Springer Science+Business Media New York 2013

Solution

In this case, the dead space in the Butterfly needle filled with succinylcholine from the last injection was the cause of the bradycardia. The injection of meperidine pushed the succinylcholine into the vein before the meperidine. This last dose of succinylcholine thus became a second dose. The dead space of a Butterfly needle has been reported at approximately 0.3 ml. Giving atropine, 0.1 mg, reverses the bradycardia, and the case proceeds uneventfully.

Discussion

Equipment dead space has been shown to be a hazard [1]. In a study by Macfie [2], the dead spaces of various cannulae, syringes, and epidural catheters were measured by displacing the dead space volume with water and measuring the weight gain. He found that 10–30 % of a 1-ml IV dose will remain in the dead space, depending on the type and gauge of the cannulae. The dead space of an epidural catheter was approximately 1 ml.

Recommendation

To avoid the complication reported here, all cannulae should be flushed with normal saline to ensure that no drug is retained in the dead space.

References

1. Wilson ME, Mayor AH. Suxamethonium in a cannula deadspace—a danger. Anaesthesia. 1991;46:599–600.
2. Macfie AG. Equipment deadspace and drug administration. Anaesthesia. 1990;45:145–7.

Chapter 35
Case 35: Hypotension on Induction of Anesthesia in a Trauma Patient

A 12-year-old boy (50 kg) is admitted to the emergency room after a fall of 30 m while climbing in the local mountains. On admission he is pale, drowsy but conscious, and oriented for time and place. On examination, multiple abrasions are found all over his body. A large hematoma is found on the back of his head. His neurologic examination is normal. He has a compound fracture dislocation of his right ankle. His upper lumbar vertebrae are tender and so is the front of his sternum, but rib springing is pain free. His vital signs are stable (pulse 96 beats per minute (bpm), sinus rhythm, blood pressure [BP] 110/70, and hematocrit [Hct] 30 %). An intravenous (IV) line is started and crystalloids given. His chest and skull X-rays are normal. A compression wedge fracture of the body of the tenth thoracic vertebrae is found. The surgeon wants to proceed with internal fixation of the ankle fracture, and the patient is taken to the operating room. After all monitors are placed on the child, anesthesia is induced with a rapid-sequence technique consisting of ketamine, 75 mg, and succinylcholine, 80 mg. A 6-mm cuffed oral endotracheal tube (ETT) is inserted into the trachea and the lungs ventilated via a Narkomed 2B machine. The tidal volume is 500 ml. Shortly after induction of anesthesia, with no change in electrocardiogram (ECG) shape and form, the BP rapidly falls to 40 mmHg but the pulse remains unchanged. No other drugs have been given. The chest is seen to expand equally, and bilateral air entry is good, with no evidence of bronchospasm. The inflation pressure remains unchanged, there is no cutaneous manifestation of any allergy, and no abdominal distension is seen.

Question

You give incremental doses of phenylephrine with some improvement in BP; however, the BP continues to decrease. The end-tidal CO_2 trace is measurable but low (values of 20 mmHg are recorded). What is the likely cause of this hypotension and what will you do now?

J.G. Brock-Utne, *Near Misses in Pediatric Anesthesia*,
DOI 10.1007/978-1-4614-7040-3_35, © Springer Science+Business Media New York 2013

Solution

Cardiac tamponade should always be considered in these cases. The surgeon should be informed and asked to help. In this case, the surgeon performed an upper midline laparotomy, which revealed a bulging inferior pericardium. When the pericardium was incised, a gush of 100 ml of dark blood and clot was released. There was an immediate increase in both pulse rate and arterial BP. The patient had an uneventful postoperative course and was discharged home after 8 days.

Discussion

The only important factor in the diagnosis of cardiac tamponade during anesthesia is a high index of suspicion. As in this case, the only sign present was hypotension. Symmes and Berman [1] state that in a case of cardiac tamponade, all of the common features of cardiac tamponade may be absent. The common features are an increase in pulse, pulsus paradoxus, hypotension, elevated jugular venous pulse, friction rub, Kussmaul's sign, and decreased heart sounds. In this case, the pulse remained unchanged at 90 bpm despite severe hypotension. However, bradycardia has been observed during acute tamponade in anesthetized dogs [2]. These authors suggest that the sinoatrial node may be rendered ischemic, causing the shift of the pacemaker with a resultant bradycardia. Indeed, bradycardia may be protective in these cases as it prevents myocardial damage by allowing longer ventricular filling when the preload is decreased [3]. Vagal slowing from acute blood loss has also been reported in hypotensive patients. Blood transfusion not only restores BP, it also causes an increase in heart rate [4].

Other causes of sudden hypotension such as a concealed large hemorrhage, pneumothorax, or acute anaphylaxis must also be considered. In this case, a compression fracture of L1 suggests major trauma and, in retrospect, a potential cardiac tamponade or severe retroperitoneal bleed should have been considered. The preoperative insertion of a central venous line could have clinched the diagnosis much earlier. The sternal tenderness was minimal, but one wonders if lateral X-ray views of the sternum should always be done in these cases.

Recommendation

In cases of major trauma, it is imperative to have a high index of suspicion that a cardiac tamponade, pneumothorax, or concealed hemorrhage may suddenly occur.

References

1. Symmes JC, Berman ND. Early recognition of cardiac tamponade. Can Med Assoc J. 1977; 116:863–4.
2. Kostregva DR, Castaner A, Pedersen DH, Kampine JP. Nonvagally mediated bradycardia during cardiac tamponade or severe hemorrhage. Cardiology. 1981;68:65–79.
3. Horgan JH. Cardiac tamponade. BMJ. 1987;295:563–4.
4. Sander-Jensen K, Secher NH, Bie P, Warberg J, Schwartz TW. Vagal slowing of the heart during haemorrhage: observations from 20 consecutive hypotensive patients. BMJ. 1986;292: 364–6.

Chapter 36
Case 36: Delayed Postoperative Respiratory Obstruction

A 2-year-old boy (12 kg) is admitted as an outpatient for electroretinography under general anesthesia. His medical history is unremarkable. He underwent, uneventfully, a similar procedure under general anesthesia at the age of 6 months. He has no known allergies and is on no drug therapy. He has had a recent upper respiratory tract infection, but his preoperative physical examination is normal. He is premedicated with oral midazolam (0.07 mg/kg) with an antacid for faster onset of sedation [1]. The child is anesthetized with sevoflurane in oxygen, and an intravenous (IV) infusion is established. Atropine and vecuronium are given in usual doses, and the trachea is intubated atraumatically with a 4.5-mm internal diameter (i.d.) tracheal tube. Anesthesia is maintained with sevoflurane and nitrous oxide in 30 % oxygen. One hour later, the procedure is completed and the child is awakened from the anesthetic. The pharynx is suctioned with a soft, rubber catheter without vision and the tracheal tube is removed. The postoperative course is uneventful. Suddenly after 20 min in the recovery room, the child stands up in bed. He has an episode of choking and coughing that leads to cyanosis. He is quickly placed in the right lateral position and given oxygen 100 % via mask. The child resumes normal breathing and the oxygen saturation is now 100 %. You carefully listen to the child's chest and find no abnormality. You lift him up to show the anxious parents that there is nothing to worry about but as you do that he coughs and retches and the oxygen saturation falls to 88 %. You put the child down and he recovers again.

Question

What will you do now and what can be the cause of this desaturation?

Solution

Always remember that you must examine the throat too. When you do so, you see a large, swollen uvula. The treatment of choice is mist, nebulized racemic epinephrine, and IV dexamethasone. In a previous case report [2], it took approximately 24 h before the child's uvula was decreased to normal size. Thereafter he was discharged.

Discussion

There are many causes of uvulitis. The main causes include mechanical and thermal trauma, chemical and allergic reactions, infection, and nonallergic complement-mediated disorders. In a previous case report, a healthy 17-year-old who inhaled marijuana before general anesthesia developed an acute uvular edema that resulted in respiratory obstruction and admission to the hospital [2]. Dexamethasone was very successful in treating his edema, and he was discharged the next day. Most cases of postanesthetic uvular edema have involved adult patients [3–6]. The disconcerting fact of these cases is that the edema can develop any time from 45 min to 24 h after an anesthetic is administered.

Recommendations

1. Always examine a child's throat before anesthesia. Although, in this case, nothing abnormal was noted in the throat despite a history of upper respiratory tract infection, it is reassuring when a normal uvula and upper airway is seen prior to induction of anesthesia.
2. Should postoperative respiratory obstruction occur, always remember to examine the throat and not just the chest.
3. Uvular edema can be delayed (90 min [1]) and can get potentially worse before it gets better.
4. Treatment must be aggressive, and the child should be admitted to the intensive care unit (ICU).

References

1. Lammers CR, Rosner JL, Crockett DE, Chhokra R, Brock-Utne JG. Oral midazolam with an antacid increases the speed of onset of sedation in children prior to anesthesia. Paediatr Anaesth. 2002;12:26–8.
2. Haselby KA, McNiece WL. Respiratory obstruction from uvular edema in a pediatric patient. Anesth Analg. 1983;65:1127–8.

3. Mallat AM, Roberson J, Brock-Utne JG. Preoperative marijuana inhalation—an airway concern. Can J Anaesth. 1996;43:691–3.
4. Shulman MS. Uvular edema without endotracheal intubation. Anesthesiology. 1981;55:82–3.
5. Ravindran R, Priddy S. Uvular edema, a rare complication of endotracheal intubation. Anesthesiology. 1978;48:374.
6. Seigne TD, Felske A, DelGiudice PA. Uvular edema. Anesthesiology. 1978;49:375–6.

Chapter 37
Case 37: An Abnormal Capnogram

A 7-year-old boy (41 lb) (American Society of Anesthesiologists physical status I [ASA 1]) is scheduled for an emergency appendectomy. The patient has had no previous anesthesia/surgery, and his family history is negative for anesthesia-related complications. General anesthesia is induced, and after the child is asleep, the trachea is intubated. Positive pressure ventilation is then instituted using the ventilator on the anesthesia machine. Both the initial end-tidal CO_2 value (40 mmHg) and the capnograph tracing are within normal limits, with an inspiratory CO_2 of zero. Anesthesia is maintained using meperidine and vecuronium with isoflurane and nitrous oxide in oxygen. Approximately 20 min into the case, the inspired end-tidal CO_2 increases and the capnogram is noted to be abnormal (Fig. 37.1). The CO_2 absorbent canister is visually inspected. The upper compartment has a slightly bluish cast, and no color change is seen in the bottom compartment to indicate exhaustion of the CO_2-absorbent granules. Other causes of the abnormal tracing are sought. The expiratory and inspiratory valves are examined and changed without improvement in the capnogram. Rebreathing continues to be apparent. The patient's vital signs remain stable with a normal blood pressure (BP) and heart rate and 100 % oxygen saturation.

J.G. Brock-Utne, *Near Misses in Pediatric Anesthesia*,
DOI 10.1007/978-1-4614-7040-3_37, © Springer Science+Business Media New York 2013

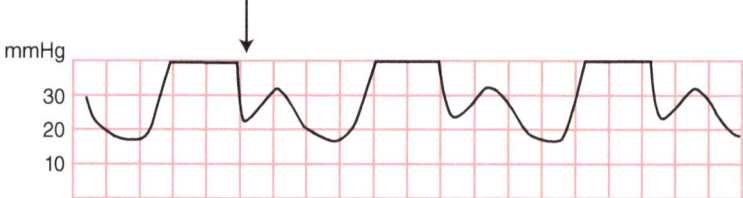

Fig. 37.1 Capnogram tracing after approximately 20 min. Note the increase in inspired end-tidal CO_2. Reprinted with permission from Pond D, Jaffe RA, Brock-Utne JG. Failure to detect CO_2 absorbent exhaustion. Seeing and believing. Anesthesiology April 2000; 92(4);1196–11971

Questions

Are you concerned and, if so, what will you do? If there is a problem, what could the cause be?

Solution

You call for a new anesthesia machine. While you wait, you increase the fresh gas flow and manually ventilate the patient. There is some improvement in the capnogram. After you attach the new anesthesia machine, the end-tidal CO_2 capnogram is again normal. The operation is concluded uneventfully, and the patient is transported to the postanesthesia care unit (PACU), with stable vital signs. You now examine the initial machine and the source of the problem is identified as exhausted CO_2 absorbent in both compartments. The dye indicator reaction in the lower compartment was obscured by the yellow discoloration of the plastic canister producing the appearance of fresh white CO_2 absorbent in the bottom canister.

Discussion

Chemical neutralization of CO_2 by absorbent granules is the method of eliminating CO_2 from an anesthetic breathing system. Neutralization of CO_2 is achieved by a chemical reaction with water and alkaline hydroxides in the granules. The reaction results in the formation of carbonic acid. Accumulation of carbonic acid results in the lowering of the pH of the granules and changes in the color of the pH-sensitive dye (ethyl violet) to violet blue. The color change is readily apparent on visual inspection. Each absorber unit contains two interchangeable transparent canisters (compartments) that are filled with absorbent. In this case, the color change was not detected because of the yellowing of the transparent plastic absorbent canisters. The yellowed plastic, which is filtered out the blue/violet wavelengths, gives the granules the appearance of the original white color. It was not until opening the canisters that the intensely purple color of completely exhausted absorbent was discovered. This case is similar to a case we have previously described in an adult [1].

The expected capnogram tracing resulting from exhausted CO_2 absorbent is seen in Fig. 37.2 [2]. Our tracing had an additional second peak for which we propose the following explanation: On inspiration (indicated with an arrow in Fig. 37.1), gas

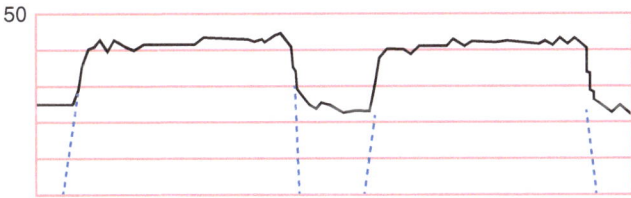

Fig. 37.2 Computer-assisted capnogram analysis showing the expected capnogram tracing resulting from exhausted CO_2 absorbent. Reproduced with permission from Genderingen HR, Gravenstein N, Gravenstein JS. Computer assisted capnogram analysis. J Clin Monit. 1987;3:198–2022

enters the inspired limb from two sources—namely, fresh gas flow from the anesthesia machine and gas from the bottom of the canister. The dip in the trace seen on inspiration is most likely due to dilution of the fresh gas flow with saturated CO_2 from the canisters. It is important to remember that nearly depleted soda lime can regain white/yellow color when not used for many hours. When used again, however, the soda lime very quickly becomes exhausted, leading to the problem described in this case.

Remember that with an exhausted CO_2 absorbent at fault, the high fresh gas flow rate should markedly decrease or eliminate the amount of CO_2 rebreathing [2]. If the problem is an incompetent expiratory valve, increasing the fresh gas flow will minimally affect the amount of CO_2 observed [2].

Recommendation

When an abnormal capnogram occurs with an increased inspired end-tidal CO_2, increase fresh gas flow and change the CO_2 absorbent even if it does not look to be exhausted. If changing the absorbent does not help, change the anesthesia machine.

References

1. Pond D, Jaffe RA, Brock-Utne JG. Failure to detect CO_2 absorbent exhaustion. Seeing and believing. Anesthesiology. 2000;92(4):1196–7.
2. van Genderingen HR, Gravenstein N, Gravenstein JS. Computer assisted capnogram analysis. J Clin Monit. 1987;3:198–202.

Chapter 38
Case 38: Retropharyngeal Abscess

A 1-year-old girl (18 lbs.) presents with an acute retropharyngeal abscess. The child has great difficulty in swallowing. She is able to maintain a reasonable airway by holding her head in full extension with her mouth wide open (oxygen saturation 96 % on room air). Her history is unremarkable. The family history is negative for anesthesia-related complications. The patient is receiving a cephalosporin IV. Monitors are placed in the operating room. The child is very worried and will not let you examine her mouth. Fiber-optic intubation is not an option. An experienced Ear, Nose, Throat (ENT) surgeon is available with a tracheostomy set. Because the patient has her mouth wide open, you can see the uvula. She is allowed to sit forward resting her elbows on a Mayo stand. After preoxygenation for 3 min in the sitting position, a rapid-sequence induction with thiopental (25 mg) and succinylcholine (15 mg) is performed. The vocal cords are not seen due to severe swelling of the oropharynx. Despite this, you safely place a 4-mm internal diameter (i.d.) endotracheal tube (ETT) in the trachea. Anesthesia is maintained with fentanyl and sevoflurane in nitrous oxide (70 %) in oxygen. A fluctuating mass is seen bulging forward from the posterior pharyngeal wall. The abscess is incised and drained. The surgeon insists that he has made the oropharynx space larger and, hence, it is safe to extubate the patient. You are concerned and would rather leave the ETT in overnight. You state that although you got the ETT in at the start of the procedure, you may not be able to do it again if it should prove necessary. The surgeon insists that you attempt to extubate the patient. You let the cuff down and the patient can breathe around the tube.

Questions

Are you happy to take the ETT out? If you did take it out, is there anything you would want to do before extubation that may increase the patient's safety?

J.G. Brock-Utne, *Near Misses in Pediatric Anesthesia*,
DOI 10.1007/978-1-4614-7040-3_38, © Springer Science+Business Media New York 2013

Solution

A pediatric gum-elastic bougie should be inserted through the ETT before extubation. This is in anticipation of a possible reintubation. If the airway becomes compromised, the trachea can rapidly be reintubated using the bougie. This technique eliminates the need for direct laryngoscopy, fiber-optic bronchoscopy, or, worse, emergency tracheostomy.

Discussion

This case is similar to an adult case [1] in which a gum-elastic bougie was used to reintubate a patient when respiration became inadequate during the postoperative period.

In cases such as this, the gum-elastic bougie can only be used when you are sure that the neuromuscular blockade is fully reversed and that the person can breathe around an occluded ETT with cuff deflated. Bedger and Chang [2] have described the use of a jet-stylet catheter (hollow), which has the added advantage of allowing jet ventilation of the patient's lungs. Bronchial tears have been described with plastic guides and bougies when used blindly in the airway [3]. In a study comparing endotracheal intubation by direct vision with and without a gum-elastic bougie, no difference in the occurrence of postoperative sore throat and hoarseness could be detected between the two groups [4]. However, used with care, the bougie is a valuable tool when urgently securing a difficult airway [5–9].

Recommendation

When removing an ETT in cases with difficult airways and likely reintubation, do not forget the gum-elastic bougie.

References

1. Robles B, Hester J, Brock-Utne JG. Remember the gum-elastic bougie at extubation. J Clin Anesth. 1993;5:329–31.
2. Bedger Jr RC, Chang JL. A jet-stylet endotracheal catheter for difficult airway management. Anesthesiology. 1987;55:221–3.
3. Conacher ID. Instrumental bronchial tears. Anaesthesia. 1992;47:589–90.
4. Nolan JP, Wilson ME. An evaluation of the gum elastic bougie. Intubation times and incidence of sore throat. Anaesthesia. 1992;47:878–81.
5. Macintosh RR. An aid to oral intubation. BMJ. 1949;1:28.

6. Kidd JF, Dyson A, Latto IP. Successful difficult intubation. Use of the gum elastic bougie. Anaesthesia. 1988;43:437–8.
7. McCarron SM, Lamont BJ, Buchland MR, Yates AP. The gum-elastic bougie: old but still useful [letter]. Anesthesiology. 1988;65:643–4.
8. Benson PF. The gum-elastic bougie: a life saver [letter]. Anesth Analg. 1992;74:318.
9. Dogra S, Falconer R, Latto IP. Successful difficult intubation. Tracheal tube placement over a gum-elastic bougie. Anaesthesia. 1990;45:774–6.

Chapter 39
Case 39: Rising End-Tidal Carbon Dioxide

A 6-year-old boy (20 kg) is admitted to hospital with a compound fracture of his right elbow after a fall from a tree. He has had lunch 1 h before admission. His history is otherwise unremarkable. As a 3-year-old, he underwent a tonsillectomy under general anesthesia without any problem. There is no adverse family history of anesthetic complications. On examination, the child is found to be otherwise healthy. Heart rate is 100 beats per minute (bpm). There is a low-grade systolic murmur at the apex. Blood pressure (BP) is 100/60 mmHg, and the chest is clear. The patient is taken to the operating room and all monitors are placed. General anesthesia is induced with propofol, 50 mg, and succinylcholine, 20 mg. Endotracheal intubation is performed with a No. 6 cuffed endotracheal tube (ETT). Breath sounds are equal bilaterally, and gastric breath sounds are not heard. The proximal end of the ETT is attached to a Bain system using the adapter on the Narkomed 2B machine. Anesthesia is maintained with intermittent boluses of fentanyl, vecuronium, and isoflurane 0.5–1.0 %. The fresh gas flow is 6 L (4 L of nitrous oxide and 2 L of oxygen). The lungs are mechanically ventilated using the ventilator on the Narkomed machine. Over a period of 30 min, you observe a gradual increase in end-tidal CO_2 with minimal changes in vital signs. The tympanic and esophageal temperatures record a temperature of 36.1 °C. Bilateral air entry can still be heard, and no abnormal breath sounds are heard. The peak inspiratory pressure reading is 20 cm H_2O and has not changed.

Question

Are you concerned and, if so, what will you do?

J.G. Brock-Utne, *Near Misses in Pediatric Anesthesia*,
DOI 10.1007/978-1-4614-7040-3_39, © Springer Science+Business Media New York 2013

Solution

You inspect the Bain system more closely and note that the inner tubing carrying the fresh gas flow to the distal end of the system has been disconnected. You replace the Bain system with your absorber system and the case proceeds without further problems.

Discussion

The Bain system is a streamlined modification of the Mapleson D System [1–3]. In the Bain system, the fresh gas flow is delivered via an inner tube close to the connection with the ETT. Previous case reports [4, 5] have highlighted the potential problem that can occur if the inner tube is avulsed or the system has not been connected correctly. Regarding problems with the inner tube, the simplest check is to visually inspect the system. Gross avulsions or disconnects should be seen. If there is no obvious sign of problems, then deliver into the Bain system 2 L per minute flow. The plunger from a small syringe is inserted into the distal end of the outer tube, thereby occluding the inner tube. If the system is intact, the flowmeter indicator should fall. If the machine has a relief valve, it should open [6–9]. Note that if the system has side holes at the patient's end of the inner tubing, this test will not work [10]. An alternative test by Pethick [11] has also been used [7, 12, 13].

In this case, the gradual rise of end-tidal CO_2 is caused by much of the fresh gas supply being diverted into the outer tube. During inhalation, the patient therefore breathes in a mixture of the expired CO_2 and fresh gas flow.

Recommendation

A check of the Bain system before use is imperative. An observed increase in end-tidal CO_2 caused by a faulty capnogram is extremely rare. When end-tidal CO_2 increases, action must be taken to rectify the situation.

References

1. Bain JA, Spoerel WE. A streamlined anaesthetic system. Can J Anaesth. 1972;19:426.
2. Bain JA, Spoerel WE. Flow requirement for a modified Mapleson D system during controlled ventilation. Can J Anaesth. 1973;20:629.
3. Lin YC, Brock-Utne JG. Pediatric anesthesia breathing system. Pediatr Anesth. 1996;6:1–5.
4. Paterson JG, Vanhooydonk V. A hazard associated with improper connection of the Bain breathing circuit. Can J Anaesth. 1975;22:373.

5. Hannallah R, Rosales JK. A hazard connected with re-use of the Bain's circuit: a case report. Can J Anaesth. 1974;21:511.
6. Foex P, Crampton-Smith A. A test for co-axial circuits. Anaesthesia. 1977;32:294.
7. Heath PJ, Marks LF. Modified occlusion tests for the Bain breathing system. Anaesthesia. 1991;46:213–6.
8. Chard GA. Safety check for the Bain circuit. Can J Anaesth. 1984;31:487–8.
9. Jackson IJB. Tests for co-axial systems. Anaesthesia. 1988;43:1060–1.
10. Robinson S, Fisher DM. Safety check for the CPRAM circuit. Anesthesiology. 1983;59: 488–9.
11. Pethick SL. Correspondence. Can J Anaesth. 1975;22:115.
12. Petersen WC. Bain circuit. Can J Anaesth. 1978;25:532.
13. Beauprie IG, Clark AG, Keith IC, Spence D. Pre-use testing of coaxial circuits: the perils of Pethick. Can J Anaesth. 1990;37:S103.

Chapter 40
Case 40: Acute Abdomen

A 13-year-old girl (120 lbs) presents with acute colicky abdominal pain and is scheduled for an emergency appendectomy. Her history is unremarkable. The mother informs you that the onset of the pain may be related to the patient having her first menses. Neither the patient nor the immediate family has had a general anesthetic. The mother informs you that she believes that the girl's father's family has an "upset metabolism." She knows nothing more about this abnormality except to say that she is sure it has nothing to do with succinylcholine. The father is unavailable for comment. The patient is taking no medication and is classified as an American Society of Anesthesiologists physical status II (ASA 2). The patient complains of severe abdominal pain and is very nauseous. You examine the patient and nothing abnormal is detected. The abdominal wall is lax. Some rebound tenderness is noted in the right iliac fossa, but much less than would be expected from acute appendicitis. No blood analysis or urinalysis is done. The surgeon is anxious to proceed.

Questions

Are you concerned? If so, what will you do? How will you proceed with the anesthetic?

Solution

You elect to do a rapid-sequence induction using propofol and rocuronium. The patient has an uneventful anesthetic and a normal appendix is removed.

Discussion

This case illustrates several important points:

1. A family history about an "upset metabolism" should never be taken lightly. The two problems you are very interested in are succinylcholine apnea and acute intermittent porphyria. With regard to succinylcholine, it is the better part of valor to avoid its use even though the mother tells you she does not think succinylcholine is a problem. With regard to porphyria, this is the only disease for which thiopental is contraindicated. Barbiturate administration in these patients may be followed by lower motor neuron paralysis, mental disturbances, or even death. Barbiturates stimulate the enzyme delta-aminolevulinic acid synthetase, increasing the formation of porphobilinogen, leading to progressive neuropathy. Propofol [1–5], ketamine, and etomidate [6] can be used as induction agents together with morphine and meperidine (Demerol). Nitrous oxide, oxygen volatile agents, relaxants, and reversal agents can also be used.
2. You may not think this girl has an acute appendicitis. You may be right in considering acute intermittent porphyria. Menstruation can bring on the disease, and the physical examination described in this case is classic. A urine sample should be taken and left standing. It will begin to turn dark within 20 min if acute intermittent porphyria is the correct diagnosis.

Recommendations

1. If you think a specific drug or drugs may cause harm, use alternatives.
2. Talk to your surgeon about your concern with his diagnosis.

References

1. Parr MJA, Hayden-Smith J. Propofol, porphyria and epilepsy. Anaesthesia. 1990;45:594.
2. Mitterschiffthaler G, Theiner A, Hetzel H, Fuith LC. Safe use of propofol in a patient with acute intermittent porphyria. Anaesthesia. 1988;60:109–11.
3. Cooper R. Anaesthesia for porphyria using propofol. Anaesthesia. 1988;43:611.
4. McLoughlin C. Use of propofol in a patient with porphyria. Anaesthesia. 1989;62:114.
5. Haberer JP, Malthe R. Propofol in acute porphyria. Anaesthesia. 1989;44:932.
6. Rizk SF, Jacobsen JH, Silvay G. Ketamine as an induction agent for acute intermittent porphyria. Anesthesiology. 1977;46:305–6.

Chapter 41
Case 41: Difficulty in Ventilation in the Postinduction Period

A 16-year-old boy (115 kg, 165 cm) is admitted for investigation of hematuria. Other than his obesity, he has no medical problems. There is no history of drug allergy or previous general anesthesia, nor any adverse family history of anesthetic complications. On examination, the child is found to be otherwise healthy. His chest is clear. The patient is transported to the operating room after an intravenous (IV) line is placed in his right arm. He moves himself over to the operating room table, taking care to bring his gown with him. He does not want to have his gown removed due to shyness. You assess the airway as a Mallampati grade 2 with good neck mobility. A rapid-sequence induction with propfol and succinylcholine is performed. The vocal cords are seen and a size 8 oral, disposable, high-volume, low-pressure cuff is inserted into the trachea and secured. Bilateral air entry is heard and the capnogram shows end-tidal CO_2. Further muscle relaxation is given with mivacurium 0.05 mg/kg. Anesthesia is maintained with fentanyl and isoflurane (1.5 %) in nitrous oxide (70 %) in oxygen. Automatic ventilation commences with a tidal volume of 1,000 ml and respiratory rate of 8. This generates a peak pressure of 25 cm H_2O. He is pulled down the operating table and placed in lithotomy position. His buttocks lie on the edge of the table. You notice that the airway pressure has risen to 60 cm H_2O. You attempt to ventilate by hand, but it is difficult to get air into his lungs. The other vital signs remain stable, but you are concerned and ask the surgeon to put the legs down on the operating table. There is minimal improvement in peak pressures. The nerve stimulator shows that the patient is relaxed. (You check the nerve stimulator on yourself with good effect.) You pass a suction catheter down the whole length of the endotracheal tube (ETT) without any problem. The cuff on the ETT is let down with no improvement. You ascertain that your ventilator is working adequately with normal peak pressure using a "dummy lung." You exclude bronchoconstriction anaphylaxis and pneumothorax. In desperation, you change the ETT with no improvement. Throughout this whole procedure, the oxygen saturation is 94 %.

J.G. Brock-Utne, *Near Misses in Pediatric Anesthesia*,
DOI 10.1007/978-1-4614-7040-3_41, © Springer Science+Business Media New York 2013

Questions

What will you do now? What can the problem be?

Solution

To better examine the patient's chest, you attempt to take off the patient's gown. You find the gown tightly fixed around his chest. The gown's knot, behind his back, cannot be undone. You cut the front of the gown with a pair of scissors and tear the gown off him. This immediately returns the ventilation to normal. The rest of the case proceeds without incident, and the patient has an uneventful anesthetic.

Discussion

This case is similar to the one described in a 58-year-old man weighing more than 160 kg [1]. He underwent an elective hemorrhoidectomy. As the patient was pulled down on the operating room table into the appropriate position, the gown became fixed tightly around his chest. The chest expansion was severely restricted. When the gown was removed, the ventilation immediately returned to normal.

Recommendation

Always undo the back of the gown before the patient lies down on the operating table.

Reference

1. Bailin MS. Gown tie causing difficult ventilation. Anaesthesia. 1995;50:96.

Chapter 42
Case 42: Unexplained Low Oxygen Saturation

A 16-year-old boy (180 lb) is scheduled for a repair of hand tendons after an injury caused by a saw. His vital signs are stable, with a heart rate of 100 and blood pressure (BP) of 90/60. His mother thinks he has lost a considerable amount of blood. The hematocrit (Hct) is 28 %. The patient has a history of malignant hyperthermia (MH) after a general anesthetic for a hernia repair at age 2 years. At that time, a positive family history of MH was found. His medical history is otherwise unremarkable. The patient has no known drug allergies. After discussion with the mother and the boy, an interscalene block [1] is performed with 60 ml of 1 % prilocaine and 10 ml of 0.5 % bupivacaine. Sedation with midazolam, 2 mg intravenous (IV), is given before the procedure. The usual monitoring equipment is placed, including a liquid crystal temperature strip on his forehead and a tympanic ear probe. Twenty-five minutes after the interscalene block, there is a good sensory block, a sympathetic block, and an ipsilateral Homer's syndrome. The surgeon infiltrates locally 10 ml of plain 0.25 % bupivacaine and the surgery commences. The pulse oximeter shows a gradual decrease over a few minutes to a saturation of 75 %. The FIO_2 is increased to 100 % via a face mask from a "clean" anesthesia machine. The saturation remains at 75 %. The patient's other vital signs are unchanged. His temperature is normal. The breath sounds are equal bilaterally with no adventitious sounds. The respiratory rate is 14. You are concerned and take an arterial blood gas measurement from his radial line. This shows a PaO_2 of 78 mmHg and a $PaCO_2$ of 36 mmHg with a base excess of −1 mmol/l with a derived oxygen saturation of 96 %.

Question

Are you concerned and, if so, what will you do?

J.G. Brock-Utne, *Near Misses in Pediatric Anesthesia*,
DOI 10.1007/978-1-4614-7040-3_42, © Springer Science+Business Media New York 2013

Solution

Prilocaine-induced methemoglobinemia should be suspected. Samples for both methemoglobin and prilocaine levels should be done. The treatment of choice is IV methylene blue 1 % in a dose of 1.2 mg/kg IV over a 10-min period. Usually the oxygen saturation will rise into the 1990s after approximately 15–20 min. However, it can take 45–60 min before it is above 96 %. In extreme cases, blood transfusion may be considered.

Discussion

IV dyes can cause transient, apparent desaturation [2–4] (topical anesthetics [prilocaine, benzocaine, lidocaine], nitrates, and aniline dyes). Cyanosis with hemoglobin desaturation caused by methemoglobinemia is rare. It is imperative to first rule out the more common causes of hemoglobin desaturation such as airway obstruction, tension pneumothorax, cardiovascular collapse, pulmonary embolus, and so forth. Most individuals with methemoglobin levels below 30 % are asymptomatic. Between 30 % and 40 % of patients complain of headache, lethargy, and dizziness. Significant hypoxia occurs above 60 %, and levels higher than 70 % are frequently lethal. The pulse oximetry usually indicates desaturation, with methemoglobin levels below 1 %. Pulse oximetry is an unreliable indicator of hemoglobin saturation in the presence of elevated methemoglobin levels. The pulse oximeter uses only two wavelengths of light and uses an associated algorithm to determine arterial oxygen saturation. Methemoglobin has an absorption spectrum that overlaps with that of both oxyhemoglobin and deoxyhemoglobin. As a result, the pulse oximeter will indicate a desaturation that does not accurately reflect the true degree of hemoglobin desaturation. Laboratory co-oximetry, which reads light absorbency at various wavelengths, can detect the true fraction of oxygenated hemoglobin. The arterial blood gas will show a high oxygen partial pressure in the presence of a low saturation, indicating the presence of dyshemoglobinemia. The development of induced methemoglobinemia in anemic patients can have serious effects on oxygen delivery.

Methemoglobinemia can also be inherited. Hemoglobin M is a congenital abnormality of the hemoglobin structure. It is an autosomal dominant trait and is usually diagnosed in infancy due to asymptomatic cyanosis. The diagnosis is made by hemoglobin electrophoreses. This disorder does not respond to normal pharmacologic intervention. The other inherited methemoglobinemia is a nicotinamide adenine dinucleotide, reduced (NADH)-methemoglobin reductase deficiency, which is an autosomal recessive trait. It is a rare enzymatic deficiency found mostly in Alaskan Indians and Eskimos.

Another clinically important, frequent cause of methemoglobinemia is topical benzocaine [5, 6]. Care should be taken not to excessively spray this agent into the oropharynx.

Recommendation

When cyanosis with hemoglobin desaturation occurs, remember to rule out common causes before considering methemoglobinemia.

References

1. Winnie AP. Interscalene brachial plexus block. Anesth Analg. 1970;49:455–6.
2. Scheller MS, Unger RJ, Kelner MJ. Effects of intravenously administered dyes on pulse oximetry readings. Anesthesiology. 1986;65:550–2.
3. Hjelm M, Son Holmdahl MII. Clinical chemistry of prilocaine and clinical evaluation of methaemoglobinaemia induced by this agent. Acta Anaesthesiol Scand. 1965;16(Suppl.):161–70.
4. Eisencraft JB. Pulse oximetry desaturation due to methemoglobinemia. Anesthesiology. 1988;68:279–82.
5. Townes PL, Geerstma MA. Benzocaine induced methemoglobinemia. Am J Dis Child. 1977; 131:697–8.
6. Collins JF. Methemoglobinemia is a complication of 20 % benzocaine spray for endoscopy. Gastroenterology. 1990;9:211–3.

Chapter 43
Case 43: Occlusion of an Endotracheal Tube in a Neonate

A prematurely born boy of 28 weeks' gestation (780 g) with respiratory distress is admitted to your neonatal intensive care unit (NICU). Routine ventilatory treatment is given with good result. On the third day, shortly after endotracheal suctioning, his respiratory parameters deteriorate. The peak pressures are seen to increase significantly, and hand ventilation confirms decreased compliance. You pass a suction catheter down the endotracheal tube (ETT), but this time you note an obstruction at the distal end of the ETT. A chest X-ray confirms the correct placement of the ETT but also shows a foreign object extending from the distal part of the ETT into the right main bronchus. Your thoracic surgical colleague says it is impossible to remove the object from the ETT with a fiber-optic bronchoscope. You know that you must remove the object.

Question

What would you suggest?

J.G. Brock-Utne, *Near Misses in Pediatric Anesthesia*,
DOI 10.1007/978-1-4614-7040-3_43, © Springer Science+Business Media New York 2013

Solution

If you apply continuous negative pressure to the proximal end of the ETT, there is a good chance that you may be able to remove the object with the ETT. A previous case report [1] indicates successful removal of a suction catheter fragment by that means; however, this is a potentially dangerous maneuver. If not done rapidly, serious collapse of the lungs may occur. To minimize the collapse, the vacuum pressure should not be higher than 40 cm H_2O. Before ETT removal, the patient should be ventilated with 100 % oxygen for up to 3 min [2].

Discussion

Tracheal obstruction is not uncommon in preterm infants on ventilators. The common causes are tracheobronchial secretions that are often bloody and thick. Obstructions have also occurred during ETT surfactant instillation [3, 4]. The obvious treatment of these cases is to replace the ETT. Fracture of suction catheters and retention within the ETT are rare. A high index of suspicion must be maintained when prolonged desaturation occurs after ETT suctioning.

Recommendation

When a foreign object causes obstruction in an ETT, consideration should be given to removing the object by applying continuous negative pressure to the proximal end of the ETT.

References

1. Meneghetti S, Trevisanuto D, Cantarutti F, Zanardo V. Tracheal tube obstruction by suction catheter fragment in a preterm baby with RDS. Paediatr Anaesth. 1996;6:163–4.
2. Kerem E, Yatsiv I, Goiten KJ. Effect of endotracheal suctioning on arterial blood gases in children. Intensive Care Med. 1990;16:95–9.
3. Nugent J, Hans H, Goldsmith J. Pulmonary care. In: Goldsmith JP, Karotkin EH, editors. Assisted ventilation of the neonate. Philadelphia: Saunders; 1981;67–80.
4. Morley CJ. Clinical experience with artificial surfactants. In: Robertson B, Ban Golde LMG, Battenburg JJ, editors. Pulmonary surfactant from molecular biology to clinical practice. New York: Elsevier; 1992;604–33.

Chapter 44
Case 44: Surgical Emphysema After a Motor Vehicle Accident

A 16-year-old boy (65 kg) is admitted to the hospital after a motor vehicle accident in which he was a passenger in the front seat. The boy was thrown toward the dashboard because he was not wearing a seatbelt. His only medical complaint is that he is partially deaf and wore a hearing aid that was lost on arrival to the hospital. He can therefore neither hear nor understand what is being said to him. His mother is there to comfort him. His ability to use sign language is poor. The patient has no history of drug allergy. On examination, the boy is found to be otherwise healthy with stable vital signs, except for a fractured right clavicle and surgical emphysema over his anterior neck and right supraclavicular fossa. There are many abrasions. Hematocrit (Hct) is 38 %, and the electrocardiogram (ECG) is normal. The chest X-ray shows a fractured right clavicle and mediastinal emphysema. The right lower lobe is collapsed. A computed tomography (CT) scan of his cervical spine and abdomen is normal. The thoracic CT scan reveals, again, air in the anterior chest wall and superior and anterior mediastinum. The thoracic surgeon diagnoses a bronchial tear that now has hopefully sealed and elects to observe him in the intensive care unit (ICU). Initially he does well, but on the third day after admission he becomes febrile and develops a productive cough. You take him to the operating room and induce general anesthesia. Through an endotracheal tube (ETT), the thoracic surgeon performs a fiber-optic bronchoscopy and sees no bronchial tear. The surgeon aspirates thick secretions and old blood from the right lower lobe. After this procedure, the patient improves sufficiently to be discharged 5 days later. Four days after his discharge, he arrives back in your emergency room with inspiratory stridor. He is transferred to the ICU where you meet him again. Arterial blood gas on room air is pH 7.38, PO$_2$ is 52 mm Hg, PCO$_2$ is 46 mm Hg, and base excess is −3 mmol/l. A chest X-ray reveals a small left pneumothorax and persistent mediastinal emphysema. He still does not have a hearing aid.

J.G. Brock-Utne, *Near Misses in Pediatric Anesthesia*,
DOI 10.1007/978-1-4614-7040-3_44, © Springer Science+Business Media New York 2013

Questions

What would you do? Treat it and send him home? Or do you think his inspiratory stridor has anything to do with his previous accident? If so, what would you recommend to do?

Solution

A rigid bronchoscopy is performed under general anesthesia. A midtracheal structure (most likely scar tissue) is seen approximately 3 cm below the sternal notch. This was due to the complete transection of the trachea at the time of the accident. An end-to-end repair of the trachea is performed, and the patient is discharged 1 week later.

Discussion

Although a diagnosis was made as to a possible bronchial tear, the investigation in this case, as in a previous case [1], was inadequate. It is recommended that a rigid or flexible diagnostic bronchoscopy be done *without* an ETT. If the tracheal disruption is proximal to the distal end of the ETT, it will be missed. The difficulty in diagnosis of the tracheal transection in this case was further compounded by the patient's deafness and accompanying poor speech. In Pembroke et al. [1], when the patient was questioned more closely on his final discharge from the hospital, he admitted to difficulty in breathing when turning his head from side to side.

It is important in these cases to make an early diagnosis and repair a tracheal rupture as soon as possible [2–5]. Nuclear magnetic resonance imaging may prove very useful.

Tracheal transection is usually seen approximately 2–3 cm from the carina. All or one of the following may be present: neck pain, cough, hemoptysis, subcutaneous emphysema, dysphonia, dyspnea, tachypnea, and difficulty in breathing when moving the head from side to side. The anesthetic management of these cases is with gaseous induction rather than with fiber-optic intubation. Fiber-optic intubation is more an aid to diagnoses than it is a method of securing an airway in an emergency situation.

Recommendations

1. Remember that the clinical picture of tracheobronchial disruption is not uniform.
2. Any patient with evidence of extrapulmonary air leak after trauma should have a bronchoscopy performed *without* an ETT.

References

1. Pembroke AP, Klineberg P, Johnson DC. Traumatic tracheal disruption—diagnostic difficulties (case report). Anaesth Intensive Care. 1995;23:206–7.
2. Swoboda L, Walz H, Kirchner R, Wertzel H, Hasse J. Tracheal and bronchial rupture after blunt thoracic trauma. Zentralbl Chir. 1993;118:47–52.
3. Verstraeten AF, Westermann CJ, Knaepen PJ, Vanderschueren RG. Tracheobronchial lesions after closed thoracic injuries. Rev Mal Respir. 1992;9:623–8.
4. Symbas PN, Justicz AG, Ricketts RR. Rupture of the airways from blunt trauma. Ann Thorac Surg. 1992;54:177–83.
5. Bein T, Lenhart FP, Berger H. Rupture of the trachea during difficult intubation. Anaesthesist. 1991;40:456–7.

Chapter 45
Case 45: Postoperative Respiratory Arrest

A 14-year-old boy (72 kg) with idiopathic scoliosis is scheduled for spinal instrumentation with Harrington rod placement. His history and physical examination are unremarkable. The patient has had no previous anesthesia/surgery, and his family history is negative for anesthesia-related complications. The patient is taking no medication and is classified as American Society of Anesthesiologists physical status I (ASA 1). General anesthesia is induced with propofol, fentanyl, and vecuronium after all necessary monitoring equipment is placed. After the boy is asleep, the trachea is intubated with a cuffed endotracheal tube (ETT). Breath sounds are equal bilaterally, and the ETT is securely taped. Anesthesia is maintained with isoflurane and nitrous oxide in oxygen, meperidine, and vecuronium. A blood salvage system is used throughout the operation. During the procedure, he loses approximately 1 l of blood. One unit of directed blood is given intraoperatively. The operation proceeds uneventfully and, at the end of the surgery, the neuromuscular blockade is reversed. Spontaneous respiration returns and the patient follows commands. The ETT is removed and he is transported to the postanesthesia care unit (PACU). On arrival in the PACU, he is alert and vital signs are stable. Because his hematocrit (Hct) is 30 %, the surgeons ask that you to retransfuse the 500 ml of salvaged blood cells.

Approximately 20 min later, you come back to the PACU. You note that the transfusion of the salvaged blood is complete; however, you also note that the boy is hardly breathing. His oxygen saturation is 88 % and falling, and the heart rate has increased from 82 to 110 beats per minute (bpm). The blood pressure (BP) is 100/60 mmHg. You immediately commence artificial ventilation with a face mask using a Jackson Rees modification of the Ayres T-piece with 100 % oxygen. His oxygen saturation comes up to 100 %.

Questions

What will you do next? What can be the cause of the respiratory arrest?

J.G. Brock-Utne, *Near Misses in Pediatric Anesthesia*,
DOI 10.1007/978-1-4614-7040-3_45, © Springer Science+Business Media New York 2013

Solution

The nerve stimulator shows that the boy is completely relaxed. You reassure the boy and give him another dose of neostigmine and glycopyrrolate with good effect. The reason for this dilemma can be attributed to the retransfusion of the cell saver blood, which contained a sufficient amount of vecuronium to cause respiratory depression.

Discussion

Currently, two types of equipment are available for retransfusion of autologous blood: (1) the centrifuge-based cell salvage instrument in which the blood is washed and centrifuged before retransfusion as an erythrocyte concentrate and (2) the canister collection system in which the blood is collected and either concentrated and washed with standard blood bank washing instruments or transfused after filtration. These systems reduce the risks that accompany homologous blood transfusions. However, a study [1] has shown that the collection of wound drainage blood during orthopedic surgery is associated with activation of complement and release of polymorphonuclear elastase and cytokines.

This case highlights the possibility of recurarization with cell saver blood. In a study by Montefiore et al. [2], the risk of secondary neuromuscular blockade was higher with vecuronium than with atracurium from cell saver blood. This was attributed to the organ-independent Hoffmann elimination of the latter drug. The liver and the kidney play only a minor role in the elimination of atracurium. However, these organs are the primary pathways for the elimination of atracurium's metabolites, including laudanosine.

Recommendation

The practice of giving the cell saver blood in the PACU may not be safe. If transfusion is done in the PACU, the nursing staff should be informed about the possible risk of secondary neuromuscular blockade. The infusion of cell saver blood should be completed before the patient leaves the PACU.

References

1. Arnold JP, Haeger M, Bengtson JP, Bengtsson A, Lisander B. Release of inflammatory mediators in association with collection of wound drainage blood during orthopaedic surgery. Anaesth Intensive Care. 1995;23:683–6.
2. Montefiore A, Heriche C, Clergue Y, Abdelmoumen F, Sicard JF, Olivera C, et al. Neostigmine protects against secondary neuromuscular blockade induced by retransfusion of autologous blood. Anesthesiology. 1996;85(3A):806.

Chapter 46
Case 46: Rapid Increase in Body Temperature After Induction of General Anesthesia

A 14-month-old boy is scheduled to undergo repair of a cranial dysostosis. His history is unremarkable. There is evidence of increased intracranial pressure, but no hydrocephalus. The patient has had no previous anesthesia/surgery, and his family history is negative for anesthesia-related complications. He takes no medication and has no drug allergies. He is classified as American Society of Anesthesiologists physical status I (ASA 1) with a class 2 airway. Monitors include pulse oximetry, electrocardiogram (ECG), liquid crystal temperature indicator (LCTI), noninvasive blood pressure (BP) cuff, and precordial stethoscope. The child is kept warm with two heating lamps. General anesthesia is induced via face mask using sevoflurane 1–4 % in 100 % oxygen. After the child is asleep, the LCTI on the forehead is seen to increase quickly to 41.0 °C from 36.5 °C. All other parameters are within normal limits. You are concerned and alert the surgeons and call for the malignant hyperpyrexia cart.

Question

Is there anything else you would like to do before treating the patient as a potential case of malignant hyperpyrexia?

J.G. Brock-Utne, *Near Misses in Pediatric Anesthesia*,
DOI 10.1007/978-1-4614-7040-3_46, © Springer Science+Business Media New York 2013

Solution

Remove the heating lamps away from the child.

In this case, the dramatic temperature rise was due to one of the heating lamps being placed too close to the patient's head [1]. The prescribed distance is 28 in. (71 cm).

Discussion

One should always confirm the presence of a rapidly rising temperature by also feeling the patient. In this case, the child was not very warm. Checking the temperature from other sites, including the tympanic membrane [2] and the esophagus, is imperative. The latter should be checked only after an ETT has been positioned and secured. Rectal temperature is not recommended because it gives a variable reflection of core temperature [2].

The expiration date of the dantrolene in the malignant hyperpyrexia cart must be checked before use. On one occasion, when we had to use dantrolene, we found that all the vials of dantrolene in the malignant hyperpyrexia cart had expired. When one is in a rush, it is so easy to forget to check this elementary but important fact.

Recommendation

When all other parameters are normal in a case of hyperthermia, do look for other causes. They may be closer than you think.

References

1. Claure RE, Brock-Utne JG. Liquid crystal temperature indicators—a potentially serious problem in pediatric anesthesia. Can J Anaesth. 1998;45:828.
2. Benzinger M, Benzinger TH. Tympanic clinical temperature. Fifth annual symposium on temperature. Biol Med. 1975;2089–2102.

Chapter 47
Case 47: Intraoperative "Oozing"

Today you are a volunteer faculty in a nearby university hospital. You have one senior resident and two medical students working with you. Your first case is a 3-year-old boy (10 kg) who is scheduled for removal of a Wilms' tumor (nephroblastoma). The child has no medical problems other than a large mass in the loin. There is no history of drug allergy, previous general anesthesia, or any adverse family history of anesthetic complications. On examination, the child is found to be otherwise healthy. Vital signs are stable. General anesthesia is induced via face mask using sevoflurane in 100 % oxygen after all necessary monitoring equipment is placed on the child. After the child is asleep, an intravenous (IV) line is inserted and 0.15 mg atropine and 1 mg vecuronium are administered to facilitate tracheal intubation with a 5-mm internal diameter (i.d.) endotracheal tube (ETT). Bilateral air entry is heard, and the ETT is taped. Anesthesia is maintained with sevoflurane 2 % in air and 30 % in oxygen and fentanyl. The operation starts, but surgical difficulties are encountered. Significant blood loss (250 ml) is seen. The hematocrit (Hct) has fallen from 38 % to 20 %. There is blood in the urine. You call for the father's directed blood and it arrives with an orderly. You give the blood to your resident to check and administer. You continue your discussion of airway management of children to the medical students. The blood transfusion starts and the surgeon states that he has the bleeding under control.

Approximately 15 min later, the attending surgeon looks over the drapes and says to you: "There is a lot of 'oozing' in the surgical field."

Questions

Are you concerned? What will you do?

J.G. Brock-Utne, *Near Misses in Pediatric Anesthesia*,   143
DOI 10.1007/978-1-4614-7040-3_47, © Springer Science+Business Media New York 2013

Solution

You walk up to the operating table and stop the blood transfusion. You ask your resident if he checked the blood and he says, "No, I thought you did." At that moment, the orderly comes into the room and says, "I have the right blood for you now, Doc. Sorry." This case actually happened to me, but it had a happy outcome. The patient had received approximately 75 ml of A Rh-positive blood, but he was B Rh-positive. The operation concluded and he was taken to the intensive care unit (ICU), ventilated overnight, and treated with fluids and furosemide. A central line was inserted for monitoring of the central venous pressure (CVP). Hourly urine samples were set aside in the window in the ICU to see any decrease in hematuria. By the next morning (22 h later), his urine was clear and he made an uneventful recovery.

In awake patients who get the wrong blood, the signs and symptoms of a hemolytic transfusion reaction include chills, tachycardia, hypotension, nausea, fever, urticaria, hematuria, and loin pain. In the anesthetized patient, the diagnosis of hemolytic transfusion is much more difficult. Only a high index of suspicion can save the day. Hemoglobinuria (not caused by surgery), bleeding diathesis (oozing), or an unexplained hypotension may raise the alarm. In this case, the sudden increase in oozing noted by the surgeon shortly after the blood was given was the important sign.

Discussion

The incidence of fatal hemolytic transfusion reactions (HTRs) is 1 in 300,000–700,000 red blood cell transfusions [1]. ABO-incompatible red blood cell transfusions are reported to be approximately 1 in 3,000 units [2]. The signs and symptoms of HTRs may follow as little as 10–20 ml of incompatible blood [3]. The severity of a reaction is generally proportional to the amount of the incompatible blood infused and the type of incompatibility and length of time before treatment is initiated [3]. When an acute HTR is suspected, the transfusion must be stopped and the transfusion service immediately notified. All cross-matched units must be rechecked. Treatment is directed toward the most serious sequelae—namely, acute renal failure and coagulopathy. Urine output should be maintained at a minimum of 1–2 ml/kg per hour with IV fluids, furosemide, and low-dose dopamine.

The possible transmission of hepatitis and/or human immunodeficiency virus (HIV) is the principal concern of patients and physician [4]. However, transfusion errors are 50–100 times more likely to occur than transfusion-transmitted HIV [5, 6].

Laboratory evaluations include urine and plasma hemoglobin determinations, other tests verifying hemolysis, and baseline coagulation studies.

Recommendation

An increase in oozing shortly after blood is given intraoperatively should be a warning signal that an incompatible blood transfusion may be in progress.

References

1. Linden JF, Tourault MA, Schribner CL. Decrease in frequency of transfusion fatalities. Transfusion. 1997;37:243–4.
2. Linden JV, Kaplan HS. Transfusion errors: cause and effects. Transfus Med Rev. 1994;8:169–83.
3. Benson KT, Chapin JW, Despotis GJ, et al. Questions and answers about transfusion practices. 3rd ed. Park Ridge: American Society of Anesthesiologists; 1998.
4. Krombach J, Kampe S, Gathof BS, Diefenbach C, Kasper SM. Human error: the persistent risk of blood transfusion: a report of five cases. Anesth Analg. 2002;94:154–6.
5. Linden JV, Wagner K, Voytovich AE, Sheehan J. Transfusion errors in New York state: an analysis of 10 years' experience. Transfusion. 2000;40:1207–13.
6. Schreiber GB, Busch MP, Kleinmann SH, Korelitz JJ. The risk of transfusion-transmitted viral infections. N Engl J Med. 1996;334:1685–90.

Chapter 48
Case 48: A Tip for Nasotracheal Intubation

You are an attending anesthesiologist in a large university hospital. Today you are to anesthetize an otherwise healthy 5-year-old boy. He is to undergo a prolonged facial maxillary surgery to correct facial bone damage caused by a motor car accident 6 months ago. The surgeon is requesting a nasal intubation and the table is turned 180°. He does not want the endotracheal tube (ETT) over the head but straight from the nose and down over the mouth and chin.

Even though there are formulas to be used to work out the required length of a nasotracheal tube [1, 2], your resident has already cut the ETT to a predetermined length, using his clinical judgment. He rightly states that increasing the length of the endotracheal tube will increase the work of breaking [3, 4].

Your resident has attached the ETT connector to the proximal end. His rationale is that if you cut the ETT after the placement of the tube, it is very difficult to get the ETT connector into the ETT as there is no ETT to hold onto.

Question

You agree with him, but ask him if there is another way to attach the ETT connector to the ETT after the ETT is placed?

Solution

After induction of anesthesia, an uncut ETT with its connector is placed nasally into the trachea. The correct placement is achieved by observing the ETT entering the trachea and by listening for bilateral chest air entry. The ETT is marked with a pen where it is to be cut outside the nose. A surgical blade or scissors are used to cut the ETT, but only 2/3 across its lumen [5] (Fig. 48.1). The tube connector is then placed in the proximal ETT by holding the "proximal handle." The "handle" prevents the ETT from getting malpositioned and makes it easier to insert the connector and prevent malposition.

This procedure obviates the need to pull out the ETT in order to obtain a grip while inserting the connector. Furthermore, it prevents unnecessary length remaining outside the nares. If the ETT is too long, it can inadvertently become kinked, and its extra length outside the nose can be an annoyance to the surgeon. The technique can also be used if the nasal ETT is judged to be too long after it has been placed.

Recommendation

The technique should help get the correct length for the nasal ETT.

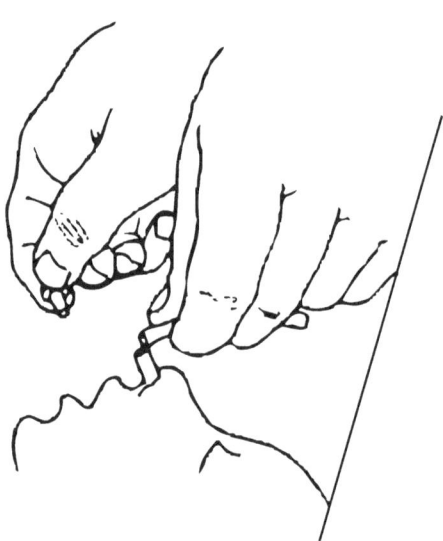

Fig. 48.1 A tip for nasotracheal intubation. Reproduced with permission from Soni AK Paes ML., Fetting the length rifght. Anaesthesia. 1994;49:549

This procedure obviates:
A. the need to pull out the tube slightly to obtain a grip while inserting the connector
B. any unnecessary length remaining outside the nares.

References

1. Coldiron JS. Estimation of nasotracheal tube length in neonates. Pediatrics. 1968;41:823–8.
2. Lau N, Playfor SD, Asrar R, Dhanarass M. New formulae for predicting tracheal tube length. Paediatr Anaesth. 2006;16:1238–43.
3. Playfor SD. New formula for predicting tracheal tube length. Paediatr Anaesth. 2007;17:711.
4. Galante D, Pellico G. New formula for predicting tracheal tube length. Paediatr Anaesth. 2007;17:710.
5. Soni AK, Paes ML. Getting the length right. Anaesthesia. 1994;49:549.

Chapter 49
Case 49: A Case of Anisocoria Following General Anesthesia

A 12-year-old boy (American Society of Anesthesiologists physical status II [ASA 2]) (62 kg and 5′) is scheduled for a repair of a pectus excavatum (funnel chest). His preoperative laboratory values and chest X-ray are normal. After adequate sedation with oral midazolam (0.07 mg/kg), you take him to the operating room where an intravenous (IV) line is placed. Routine general anesthesia is induced using propofol, fentanyl, and vecuronium. The airway is secured and anesthesia maintenance is with N_2O/O_2 with sevoflurane. Another IV is placed together with a right radial arterial line. Attempts to cannulate the right internal jugular vein (IJV) prove difficult, as the ultrasound machine intermittently stops working. A new ultrasound machine is brought in and the IJV is successfully cannulated.

Fourteen hours later, the boy is in the intensive care unit (ICU). He is extubated, and his vital signs are stable. His pain level is 2–3. The ICU nurse notices anisocoria of the right pupil (2 mm) compared to the left (4 mm). Both pupils react briskly to light, but the right pupil dilates poorly under conditions of dim illumination (dilatational lag). You are called and confirm the findings but also note a 1–2 mm ptosis on the right. There are no other abnormal ocular or neurological signs. You call for an ophthalmic consult, but you are told he will not be able to get there before next morning.

Questions

What is the diagnosis? Is there a simple test you would suggest to make the diagnosis while you wait for the ophthalmologist?

J.G. Brock-Utne, *Near Misses in Pediatric Anesthesia*,
DOI 10.1007/978-1-4614-7040-3_49, © Springer Science+Business Media New York 2013

Solution

1. Acquired Horner's syndrome.
2. Dripping cocaine (4 %) in the right eye. If there is no dilation of the pupil, then the patient has an acquired Horner's syndrome.

Discussion

Damage to the oculosympathetic pathway following the IJV insertion is an unusual cause of Horner's syndrome. In a previous case report [1], the Horner's syndrome had not gone away at 7 months. Fortunately, the boy had no symptoms from the Horner's and was only minimally concerned about its cosmetic effect. In another case report [2], the anisocoria was still present 5 weeks later but much improved after IJV insertion.

Recommendation

When your ultrasound machine does not function properly—stop, wait, and get a new one.

References

1. Talks SJ, Shah P, Sinha PA. Horner's syndrome following central line insertion. Anaesthesia. 1994;49:553.
2. Ford S, Lauder G. Case report of Horner's syndrome complicating internal jugular venous cannulation in a child. Paediatr Anaesth. 2007;17:396–8.

Chapter 50
Case 50: A Routine Tonsillectomy and Adenoidectomy

A 7-year-old immigrant boy is admitted for removal of tonsils and adenoids (T-A). The child was born at full-term delivery but needed tracheal intubation and suction at birth. He has always been a poor feeder and gets asthma attacks regularly. Despite that, according to the mother, he was doing well until after his arrival in the USA, 4 months ago. Since coming here, his asthma has worsened. He often gets severe episodes of coughing and vomiting and becomes tachypnoeic, tachycardic, and cyanotic. He also has had two episodes of pneumonia for which he was admitted to the hospital.

On exam, he is small for his age. With the exception of his lungs that are slightly wheezy, his exam is normal. Since he has no fever, it is decided to go ahead with the procedure.

The child is taken to the operating room and adequately sedated with oral midazolam. An intravenous (IV) line is established and a routine IV induction ensues with propofol and rocuronium. Laryngoscopy showed a normal supraglottic airway. A #6 endotracheal tube (ETT) with cuff is passed atraumatically into the trachea, and the cuff is inflated just below the vocal cords. Bilateral air entry is heard and end-tidal CO_2 is seen.

However, it is impossible to obtain an adequate seal (for ventilation) despite inflating the functioning ETT cuff. You confirm that the ETT is in the trachea but you now see a lot of secretions in the back of the pharynx that seem to be bubbling during inspiration.

You suspect a possible tracheoesophageal fistula (TEF).

There is still bilateral air entry and end tidal CO_2. The vital signs are stable but the O_2 saturation has fallen from 97 % to 92 %. The patient is fully paralyzed and asleep.

Question

What will you do now?

J.G. Brock-Utne, *Near Misses in Pediatric Anesthesia*,
DOI 10.1007/978-1-4614-7040-3_50, © Springer Science+Business Media New York 2013

Solution

This happened to me and I let the cuff down, advanced the ETT further down into the trachea, and blew up the cuff. Luckily I got a seal. The operation was abandoned.

A few days later, the patient underwent a repair of an H-type TEF. Six months later, the symptoms of asthma had disappeared.

Discussion

TEFs are usually diagnosed in the neonatal period with a triad consisting of coughing associated with feeding, gaseous distention of the stomach, and asthma or recurrent chest infections. TEF can also be diagnosed later [1, 2] as an outpatient or diagnosed when the child is admitted to an ICU for intermittent positive pressure ventilation. In these cases, distention of the stomach can be a telling sign [2].

Recommendation

Always be aware of any child presenting with asthma-like symptoms and recurrent unexplained pulmonary pneumonia/aspiration. They may have an undiagnosed TEF.

References

1. Frates C, terMeulen DC, Yee WF. Congenital tracheoesophageal fistula (H-type) in a six year old. Clin Pediatr. 1990;29:117–9.
2. Teasdale AR, Nielsen MS. Late presentation of tracheoesophageal fistula. Anaesthesia. 1994;49:307–8.

Chapter 51
Case 51: Drug Overdose

A 16-year-old girl is admitted to the emergency room (ER) following an overdose of unknown drugs and amount. Her parents tell you that she has been depressed after a breakup with her boyfriend. She is otherwise healthy but has been taking antidepressants for about 4 weeks; the parents cannot recall what they are called. Although she is asymptomatic, gastric lavage is performed in the ER and activated charcoal is instilled into her stomach.

She is kept in the ER for observation. Unfortunately over the next 2 h the girl becomes progressively drowsier. You are called to secure the airway.

You examine the patient. Charcoal is visible on her lips and tongue. After reviewing the chart and routine laboratory results you declare her an ASA 1E (American Society of Anesthesiologists physical status I emergency). The anesthesia equipment including the laryngoscope is working.

Questions

Are there any concerns prior to doing an RSII (rapid sequence induction and intubation) in this patient in the ER?

If so, what?

Solution

Turn off the ambient light in the ER prior to RSII.

Discussion

In a previous case [1], after an RSII, laryngoscopy was performed; gross charcoal staining of the entire upper airway was seen. Despite a good light from the laryngoscope, everything was black. It was virtually impossible to see the laryngeal inlet. The very limited light reflection was compounded by the "superb" ambient lighting in the ER. In the previously reported case [1], the recommendation was to turn off the ambient lighting prior to RSII, thereby allowing a degree of dark adaption to occur.

Attempting to intubate in bright sunlight can be very difficult. I know from personal experience in Africa. Dr. van der Heyden, a German doctor I was working with in Zululand, taught me that in those cases always secure the airway by covering your head and that of the patient's with a dark blanket. Dark adaption does make securing the airway easier.

Recommendation

Activated charcoal can make what seems an easy intubation, difficult. Always turn off operating room (OR) or ER lights a few minutes prior to induction. Have a blanket ready to cover yours and the patient's heads. A fiber-optic intubating scope and other airway devices should always be readily at hand.

Reference

1. Moore EW, Davies MW. A black hole: an unexpected cause of difficult intubation. Anaesthesia. 1996;51:795–6.

Chapter 52
Case 52: Cardiac Arrest in a Neonate

You are an intensive care unit (ICU) pediatric attending called to assist with a cardiac arrest in a neonate. The infant has just been brought back to the ICU following a repair of tracheoesophageal atresia. The patient's history, physical examination, and laboratory results (30 min before arrival in the ICU) were all within normal limits.

The child has been left intubated with 3.0 endotracheal tube (ETT) postoperatively as he is cold (34.5 °C). Just before the cardiac arrest, the child had lost his only intravenous (IV) line. The diagnosis of cardiac arrest was made by the ICU nurse based on loss of the pulse oximetry trace, ST segment depression, and a decrease in heart rate (sinus rhythm) from 138 to 98 beats per minute (bpm). The arterial blood pressure has stopped working an hour ago. Attempts to get a new one inserted have failed. The noninvasive BP reading is 40/25 mmHg. You diagnose a pulseless electrical activity (PEA). Cardiopulmonary resuscitation (CPR) is started with insufflation of 100 % oxygen. On listening to the lungs, you diagnose a right-sided pneumothorax.

You place an underwater drain rapidly [1] and order epinephrine to be given through the ETT. Your medical student hands you an atomized sprayer (MADgic, Wolfe Tory Medical Inc. Salt Lake City, UT, USA) and asks if you can use that. He tells you that MADgic has been recommended to deliver drugs further down the tracheobronchial tree rather than injecting drugs directly with a syringe at the Y-junction or into the ETT. The MADgic, he states, provides a more consistent delivery of the entire injected amount beyond the tip of the ETT.

You ignore the student and inject epinephrine into the ETT with a syringe. By using epinephrine and relieving the tension pneumothorax the neonate's vital signs are improved immediately. The child makes an uneventful recovery.

You turn to the medical student and say, "I know about the MADgic. But there are several reasons why you should not use it."

J.G. Brock-Utne, *Near Misses in Pediatric Anesthesia*,
DOI 10.1007/978-1-4614-7040-3_52, © Springer Science+Business Media New York 2013

Question

Can you think of any?

Solution

In a study [2], we found that rather than delivering the intended atomized spray of drug into the trachea the MADgic failed for the following reasons:

1. The device is not long enough to protrude at the end of the ETT (unless the ETT is cut).
2. The device will not fit into a minimum size 5 ETT.
3. The small caliber of pediatric tubes inhibits the velocity of the drug delivery, leading the drug to collect in the distal end of the tube.
4. The MADgic contains an inherent dead space. If you elect to use this device, then you must take that into account when choosing drug volume.

Added to these points above is the fact that MADgic is "off label" for pediatrics.

The study [2] concluded that injecting drugs with a syringe directly at the Y-junction or into the ETT provides a more consistent delivery of the entire injected amount beyond the tip of the ETT.

In the above case, relying on the use of MADgic during the cardiac arrest may not have had the desired effect or at best minimal effect. However, in one study the effectiveness of ETT installation of drug is rarely effective in the setting of CPR or cardiac arrest [3]. It is interesting to note that the intraosseous route has been shown to be more reliable and faster than the ETT [4].

Recommendation

Using any off-label device is not recommended.

References

1. Brock-Utne JG, Brodsky JB, Haddow G, Mark JB. A simple underwater seal apparatus for use in emergencies. J Cardiothorac Vasc Anesth. 1991;5:195–7.
2. Bernstein O, Eide AM, Brock-Utne JG. Drug delivery via the tracheal tube using an airway device. A warning. Pediatr Anesth. 2007;17:604.
3. Nieman JT, Stratton SJ. Endotracheal versus intravenous epinephrine and atropine in-out of hospital "primary" and post-countershock asystole. Crit Care Med. 2000;28:1815–9.
4. LaRocco BG, Wang HE. Intraosseous infusion. Prehosp Emerg Care. 2003;7:280–5.

Chapter 53
Case 53: Bilateral Tourniquets. Beware

Today you are anesthetizing an 18-year-old male (60 kg, 175 cm) American Society of Anesthesiologists physical status II (ASA 2) for bilateral knee arthroscopies. He has been worked up for possible cardiomyopathy. The note from the cardiologist tells you it is mild and his ejection fraction (EF) is 50 %. On physical exam, he has no heart murmurs. His electrocardiogram (EKG) shows flattened T waves and some evidence of ventricular hypertrophy. He requests no premedication. A routine general anesthetic with propofol ensues and a laryngeal mask airway (LMA) #4 is inserted with a good seal. Spontaneous breathing resumes and he is maintained on N_2O 70 % in oxygen and sevoflurane 1 % with meperidine up to 2 mg/kg. No antibiotic is given as per surgeon's preference.

Since there are two surgeons working, one fellow and one attending, both lower limbs are elevated and exsanguinated with an Esmarch bandage at the same time. Bilateral pneumatic tourniquets are applied and inflated to 300 mmHg.

Just before surgery starts, the patient's breathing becomes labored. There is prolonged expiration and the neck veins are distended. You listen and diagnose moderate to severe bronchospasm. His saturation falls from 100 % to 89 % and the heart rate increases from 72 to 97 beats per minute (bpm). His blood pressure (BP) is cycling. You remove the LMA and ventilate with O_2 100 % and sevoflurane 3 %. Unfortunately, there is no improvement in his vital signs. You give 100 mcg of epinephrine IV—still no improvement.

Question

Before you administer more epinephrine, what will you do?

J.G. Brock-Utne, *Near Misses in Pediatric Anesthesia*,   161
DOI 10.1007/978-1-4614-7040-3_53, © Springer Science+Business Media New York 2013

Solution

In a previous case, both tourniquets were let down and the bronchospasm resolved within 1–2 min [1].

Discussion

Bronchoconstriction can be mediated via vagal afferents (J-receptors). The receptors respond to pulmonary congestion and increased pulmonary capillary pressure. This can occur in left ventricular failure or fluid overload. In this case [1], substantial autotransfusion was thought to be the cause of the bronchospasm with a concurrent rise in central venous pressure (CVP). The latter seen by the distended neck veins. A subsequent increase in pulmonary capillary pressure may have caused activation of the J-receptors resulting in overt bronchospasm. By letting the tourniquet down, the bronchospam improved. It is well documented that in acute pulmonary edema there can be bronchospasm. Although there was no evidence that this patient was in pulmonary edema, the author [1] argues that a state of subclinical left ventricular failure was in fact present and that the bronchospasm was the only clear manifestation.

It is interesting to note that in the above case, the procedure was not abandoned and both tourniquets were again reinflated. Again bronchospasm occurred but the surgery carried on. Some improvement was seen when one tourniquet was deflated. Complete resolution of the bronchospasm was seen when the last tourniquet was deflated.

Bilateral lower limb tourniquets are known to cause arterial hypertension [2], and dangerous intracranial pressure (ICP) increases can occur both during inflation and deflation of the tourniquet. During reperfusion of the ischemic limbs, there is an increase in $PaCO_2$ [3, 4].

Recommendation

Remember that bronchospasm can be caused by the inflation of tourniquets.

References

1. Sammut MS. Bronchospam followed application of bilateral lower limb tourniquets. Anaesthesia. 1991;46:509–10.
2. Kaufman RD, Walts LF. Tourniquet-induced hypertension. Br J Anaesth. 1982;54:333–6.
3. Eldridge PR, Williams S. Effect of tourniquet on cerebral perfusion pressure in head-injured patients. Anaesthesia. 1989;44:973–4.
4. Townsend HS, Goodman SB, Schurman DJ, Hackel A, Brock-Utne JG. Tourniquet release: systemic and metabolic effects. Acta Anaesthesiol Scand. 1996;40:1234–7.

Chapter 54
Case 54: Neurofibromatosis. A Warning

A 16-year-old boy was diagnosed with neurofibromatosis (NF) at the age of 14 because of rapidly progressive weakness and wasting of his right arm. A magnetic resonance imaging (MRI) at the time showed multiple NF from C4-7.

Four months previously, he underwent a cervical laminectomy (C4-T1) and anterior fusion from C3-T1. He made a good recovery. But he still had the residual hand muscle weakness and wasting of both thenar and hypothenar eminences. He was admitted this time for tendon transfers to his right hand.

Speaking to him and his parents, the boy claimed he felt fine with no neck problems.

On exam, he was otherwise healthy with a Mallampati grade 1. The neck extension was reduced to 50 % of normal. Otherwise, the exam was normal.

A lateral cervical spine X-ray done 5 months ago only showed the previous fusion.

Question

In this case, would you repeat the cervical spine X-ray or are you happy to proceed without one?

J.G. Brock-Utne, *Near Misses in Pediatric Anesthesia*,
DOI 10.1007/978-1-4614-7040-3_54, © Springer Science+Business Media New York 2013

Solution

In a case [1], the patient was anesthetized without a preoperative cervical spine X-ray. The patient received a routine general anesthetic with a laryngeal mask airway (LMA). Postoperatively, he was fine and had no complaints. On the second day after the surgery, he complained of a sore neck. He was examined and there were no sensory or neurological deficits. A cervical spine X-ray was ordered and showed: "A grossly unstable dislocation at C4-5." He then admitted that he had heard a "loud crack" in his neck a few weeks before.

Discussion

Neurofibromatosis cases are not routine cases. All these patients should have a routine cervical spine X-ray. This is especially important if they have had previous cervical surgery.

A serious injury to the spinal cord could have occurred if this patient had been paralyzed and intubated.

Recommendation

All patients with neurofibromatosis should have a routine cervical spine X-ray and especially if they have had previous cervical surgery.

Reference

1. Lovell AT, Alexander R, Grundy EM. Silent, unstable, cervical spine injury in multiple neuro-fibromatosis. Anaesthesia. 1994;49:453–4.

Chapter 55
Case 55: A Machine Failure

A 16-year-old boy (American Society of Anesthesiologists physical status I [ASA 1], weight 60 Kg and height 5'7") was scheduled for a knee arthroscopy. He was the first case of the day. The anesthesia machine passed the daily checks, using the machine's electronic system. The breathing circuit was manually checked using the thumb-occlusion test. The patient was pre-oxygenated. The reservoir bag was seen to move appropriately with inspiration and expiration. Anesthesia was induced with propofol and when there was no response to the jaw thrust, a laryngeal mask airway—LMA—Unique (Laryngeal Mask Company Ltd., San Diego, CA)—was inserted without difficulty. However, manual ventilation was not possible. The reservoir bag remained empty despite closing the adjustable pressure limiting (APL) valve and activating the oxygen flush. The oxygen pipeline pressure was 50 psi. An Ambu bag (Ambu, Copenhagen, Denmark) was used to ventilate the patient. Continuous infusion of propofol kept the patient asleep. A new anesthetic machine was brought in and the operation concluded successfully.

Question

What is it that you must do prior to the faulty machine being removed from the room?

Solution

Write down the machine's number and inform your colleagues about your dilemma. Failing to do that can lead to a potential disaster.

Discussion

A friend of mine who worked in a surgery center had a similar anesthesia machine problem (described on the previous page). It occurred in the last case of the day. Luckily, the anesthetic was short and was concluded satisfactorily. He informed the charge nurse that the machine must be taken out to be serviced and a new one replaced by the morning. This was because all four rooms were to be used the next day. The next day my pal was working in a different room. All anesthetic machines in the surgery center were of the same make and model. After having put the first patient of the day asleep, the same problem recurred. Again, the Ambu bag came to the rescue. The surgery was completed uneventfully. My pal requested a new machine, only to be told there were none. In short, last night's charge nurse had simply switched the two anesthesia machines, as she did not have a reserve. Had my friend taken the faulty machine number, he would have discovered the next day that the machine he was about to use was the one he had declared faulty. Failure to ventilate with modern anesthesia workstations have been described [1].

When working in surgical centers, there are two main problems. There is limited bioengineering presence and very often no extra anesthesia machine.

Recommendation

Always make sure you identify a faulty machine. Failure to do that could prove disastrous.

Reference

1. Hilton G, Moll V, Zumaran A, Jaffe RA, Brock-Utne JG. Failure to ventilate with the Dräger Apollo anesthesia workstation. Anesthesiology. 2011;114:1238–40.

Chapter 56
Case 56: A Severe Case of Bronchospasm

You have just anesthetized a 17-year-old boy (American Society of Anesthesiologists physical status I [ASA 1], weight 70 kg, height 5′11′′) for a knee arthroscopy. Mask ventilation was easy. You placed a #7 endotracheal tube (ETT) (high volume low pressure tube) atraumatically in his trachea and inflated the cuff with 5 ml of air. To your dismay, when you attempted to manually ventilate you discover there was severe bronchospasm bilaterally. The peak pressures are over 50 cm H_2O.

You remembered from your residency that if the ETT is too far down the trachea, it can "tickle" the carina and cause bronchospasm. You pulled the ETT back to 22 cm from 24 cm at the teeth, but there was no improvement.

You passed a suction catheter, but it did not seem to go through the whole length of the ETT and stopped at about 28 cm. Obviously there was no reason to give any bronchodilators, as there seemed to be a mechanical obstruction within the ETT.

Question

Besides taking the ETT out and reintubating with another, what else would you suggest and what can the problem be?

Solution

Let the cuff down.

Discussion

Immediately there is an improvement as you have diagnosed the cuff has herniated into the lumen of the ETT [1]. This was very common when in the old days we used red rubber tubes (high pressure low volume). These tubes were autoclaved and reused again and again. With all the autoclaving, the rubber became softer and softer. Eventually, when inflating the cuff, it would herniate into the ETT. This can also occur with the modern high volume low pressure tubes [1, 2]. This is most commonly seen some time after initiation of anesthesia when there is a sudden inability to ventilate. The main reason for this delayed obstruction is the slow expansion of the cuff with N_2O [3–6]. When using an ETT, the lowest cuff pressure must be maintained to prevent leakage. Cuff pressures greater than 30 cm H_2O (22 mmHg) compress mucosal capillaries and impair blood flow. Pressures above 50 cm H_2O (37 mmHg) produce total occlusion [7, 8]. Obviously kinking of the ETT in the trachea can occur and could have been the cause in the above case. This has been reported [9].

Recommendation

When faced with a case of bronchospasm during anesthesia, always pull the ETT back and suction the ETT. If there seems to be an obstruction in the lower end of the ETT, try letting the cuff down.

References

1. Gliech SJ, Nicholson WT, Jacobs TM, Hofer RE, Sprung J. Inability to ventilate while using a silicone-based endotracheal tube. J Clin Anesth. 2008;20:389–92.
2. Ng TY, Kirimli BI. Hazards in use of anode endotracheal tube: a case report and review. Anesth Analg. 1975;54:710–4.
3. Grime PD, Tyler C. An obstructed airway: cuff herniation during nasotracheal anaesthesia for a bimaxillary osteotomy. Br J Oral Maxillofac Surg. 1991;29:14–5.
4. Patterson KW, Keane P. Missed diagnosis of cuff herniation in a modern nasal endotracheal tube. Anesth Analg. 1990;71:563–4.
5. Oyzo C, Demir K. Life-threatening complication of recurrent laryngeal nerve monitoring with EMG reinforced silicone ETT. J Craniofac Surg. 2011;22:2419–21.

6. Ward CF, Gamel DM, Benumof JL. Endotracheal tube cuff herniation: a cause of delayed airway obstruction. Anesth Analg. 1978;57:114–6.
7. Guyton D, Banner MJ, Kirby RR. High-volume, low pressure cuffs. Are they always low pressure? Chest. 1991;100:1076–81.
8. Seegobin RD, van Hasselt GL. Endotracheal cuff pressure and tracheal mucosal blood flow: endoscopic study of effects of four large volume cuffs. BMJ (Clin Res Ed). 1984;288:965–8.
9. Leissner KB, Ortega R, Bodzin AS, Sekhar P, Stanley GD. Kinking of an endotracheal tube within the trachea: a rare cause of endotracheal tube obstruction. J Clin Anesth. 2007;19:75–6.

Chapter 57
Case 57: A Peanut in the Airway

A 2-year-old boy is brought into the emergency room with wheezing and stridor. The parents accompanying the child tell you that they are sure there is a peanut stuck in his windpipe. This happened 3–4 h prior to admission. The time is now 6 p.m. Chest exam exhibits classical laryngeal obstruction and with decreased bilateral air entry. The child is frightened and very distressed. He will not have any noninvasive monitors put on, including the oxygen saturation. You are comforted by the fact that he does not look cyanosed. He is using his accessory muscles and everyone can hear that he is wheezing with each forced exhalation.

The emergency physician would like a chest X-ray but the ENT surgeon says, "Forget about that. We need to go to the operating room ASAP." With that he picks up the child and marches off to the operating suite.

Questions

You as the anesthesiologist follow along but wonder what the rush is all about. Does the surgeon have a party to go to or is there something you do not know?

Why is the ENT surgeon treating this as a real airway emergency?

J.G. Brock-Utne, *Near Misses in Pediatric Anesthesia*,
DOI 10.1007/978-1-4614-7040-3_57, © Springer Science+Business Media New York 2013

Solution

Peanuts, being an organic matter and very salty will absorb water, swell, and cause a sudden airway obstruction. Furthermore, peanuts will also cause inflammation of the airway and exacerbate the obstruction.

I have personally seen such a case in the AG Kahn hospital in Durban, South Africa [1]. The ENT surgeon Dr. Naidu carried the child up to the operating room from the emergency room. After having placed the child on the operating table, there was a sudden onset of cyanosis with several episodes of stress coughing. Inhalation induction with halothane in 100 % oxygen commenced. Spontaneous breathing became labored. Both the oxygen saturation and heart rate fell from 96 % to 89 % and 140 beats per minute (bpm) to 100 bpm, respectively. The child had become limp; Dr. Naidu without any lidocaine topicalization quickly inserted a ridged bronchoscope. A foreign body was seen in the lower end of the trachea. With the small straight metal suction, he applied negative pressure to the foreign body. He then quickly removed (from the trachea) both the ridged bronchoscope and the suction. Much to everyone's surprise and relief, the small peanut was removed intact.

The child made an uneventful recovery.

Discussion

This case is somewhat similar to case #43 in this book. In that case, a large foreign object that had stuck to the end of the endotracheal tube (ETT) and caused a severe obstruction and could not be removed by a fiber-optic bronchoscope. In that case, the foreign body was removed successfully by applying continuous negative pressure to the proximal end of the ETT trachea.

Foreign body aspiration is a common emergency and causes more than 300 deaths per annum in the USA. The most common age group is 1–2 year-olds [2, 3].

In a retrospective study by Ramierz-Figueroa et al. [4], it was found that of 59 children with foreign body aspiration, removal of an organic foreign body (38/59) from the airway was more successful with a rigid bronchoscope than a flexible fiber-optic bronchoscopy. When a forceps is used to grab the peanut, as compared to the Naidu technique (as described on the previous page) of suctioning, usually the peanut breaks into fragments. This leads to a prolonged intervention with often severe postoperative subglottic edema. Despite this, the use of forceps is considered a safer option [5].

In a case report of a 24-month-old boy who got a peanut in his airway [6], air trapping occurred. This was caused by the distention and narrowing of the airways during respiration.

There are two schools of thought as to how a child with a foreign body in the trachea should be managed. The instrumentation of larynx and trachea/bronchi may cause laryngospasm, coughing, bucking, arrhythmias, and hypertension. The problem can be avoided or minimized with using muscle relaxation and ventilation.

I prefer inhalational anesthetic without the use of muscle relaxation as ventilation can force the foreign body deeper into the small bronchi. This can cause a ball valve obstruction and, added to that, the foreign body may be difficult to remove [7]. Despite that, Kosloske in 1982 [8] recommended muscle paralysis and ventilation. Others [9] have indicated that, while the spontaneous breathing technique was used initially, muscle paralysis was employed after the foreign body was removed. The reason for paralyzing the patient was because of inadequate ventilation and/or laryngospasm.

Recommendation

Peanut inhalation in children is a serious airway concern. Remember that peanuts are organic and will swell, causing a sudden obstruction of the airway. Cooperation between the anesthesiologist and the ENT specialist is mandatory for a successful outcome.

References

1. Brock-Utne JG. Clinical anesthesia near misses and lessons learned. New York: Springer; 2008. Chapter 64.
2. Roberts JR, Benjamin JT, Fox S. Crunchy peanut butter: a cause of foreign body aspiration in children. Clin Pediatr. 1996;35:591–2.
3. Cataneo AJ, Reibscheid SM, Ruiz Junior RL, Ferrari GF. Foreign body in the tracheobronchial tree. Clin Pediatr. 1997;36:701–6.
4. Ramirez-Figueroa JL, Gochicoa-Rangel LG, Ramierz-San Juan DH, Vargas MH. Foreign body removal by flexible fiberoptic bronchoscopy in infants and children. Pediatr Pulmonol. 2005; 40:392–7.
5. Brloc F, Umihanic S. Tracheobronchial foreign bodies in children. Experience at ORL clinic Tuzla. 1954–2004. Int JPediatr Otorhinolaryngol. 2007;71:909–15.
6. Ho AMH, Soo G, Lee S, Chung DC, Crtichley LAH, Karmakar MK. Images in anesthesia: airway obstruction after peanut aspiration—air trapping is due to airway distention and narrowing. Can J Anesth. 2005;52:205–6.
7. Vane DV, Pritchard J, Colville CW, et al. Bronchoscopy for aspirated foreign bodies in children: experience in 131 cases. Arch Surg. 1988;123:885–8.
8. Kosloske AM. Bronchoscopic extraction of aspirated foreign bodies in children. Am J Dis Child. 1982;136:924–7.
9. Litman RS, Ponnuri J, Trogan I. Anesthesia for tracheal or bronchial foreign body removal in children: analysis of ninety-four cases. Anesth Analg. 2000;91:1389–91.

Chapter 58
Case 58: A Sprinkler Spike Lodged in a Patient's Head

A 6-year-old boy is admitted to a university medical center emergency room. He has fallen on his head and a metal sprinkler spike has penetrated his skull. The spike enters the head at an angle in the left temporal region, just above his ear. The length of the spike is 6–8 in. It is sticking straight back extending from his occipital region by at least 2 in. The computed tomography (CT) scan shows the spike is about 1 in. inside the brain. The child is lying on his right side, as the spike prevents him from lying flat or on his left side.

On examination he is awake, vital signs are within normal limits, but he complains about a pain in his head. His last meal was 4 h previously. Further exam revealed no other injuries and his heart and lungs are normal to auscultation. His airway exam shows a Mallampati 1 with good mouth opening. The child is moved carefully to the operating table where a rapid sequence induction and intubation (RSII) is planned with etomidate and succinylcholine in the right lateral position. The spike is supported by massive amount of gauze and towels.

Question

You have never done an RSII in the right lateral position. You would rather have him supine. But is there anything you can do to make that happen?

Solution

Take an orthopedic rod cutter and cut the sprinkler about 1 in. from the skin. This would make it possible to place the patient flat.

Discussion

In a previous case report, the sprinkler was cut as described above [1]. In that case, the RSII was uneventful in the supine position. The patient made a good recovery and was discharged on day 4.

Intubating a patient in the lateral position is known to result in a poor laryngoscopic view, with decreased time for successful intubation [1]. However, in a study [2] we found that the left lateral tilt had a superior laryngoscopic view, due mainly to the tongue falling out of the way.

We had a case in South Africa where an unfortunate worker fell off a scaffolding and got impaled on a rebar (a 1 × 1-in. and 8-ft long stainless steel bar). The rebar entered the chest at about 2 in. posterior to the axillary midline on the right and exited on the left side also posterior to the midaxillary line. Hanging there, he was cut down by rebar cutters and gently lowered to the ground. When attempting to place him in the ambulance, the rebar was too wide to let him get in. Again the rebar cutters were used. When he arrived with us, he was still very much alive. Bilateral hemopneumothoraxes were quickly treated, and he was taken to the operating room (OR). However, the patient with his rebar proved too wide to enter the OR suite. Professor LeRoux, the cardiothoracic surgeon, used the rebar cutter with great gusto. However, he left the left side of the rebar 2–3 ft out on that side while the right side was cut close to the skin. My attending at the time, Dr. Alison Holloway, performed a successful RSII. The rebar was pulled out in one piece. The patient tolerated the procedure well and was taken to the intensive care unit (ICU) intubated. We had expected that he had damaged his aorta or his pulmonary vessels and were ready as much as possible to deal with a major hemorrhage when the bar was removed. But as luck would have it, nothing happened. We were amazed. Three days later, he was out of ICU and left the hospital 7 days later.

There was another caveat to this case. Cutting metal so near to a patient's skin, there is always a risk that sawing metal could heat and thereby causing the patient to suffer a burn. Dr. Holloway, I recall, placed packing towels containing ice cubes around the metal before attempts were made to shorten them.

Recommendation

If you are ever faced with this dilemma, remember to cut the offending rod so you can do your job more safely. Be aware that metal when heated can cause a burn.

References

1. Rafique MB, Nesselrode R, De Armendi AJ. Difficult airway due to sprinkler spike in the head. Pediatr Anesth. 2008;18:891–2.
2. Buley RJR, Downing JW, Brock-Utne JG, Cuerden C. Right versus left lateral tilt for Caesarean section. Br J Anaesth. 1977;49:1009–14.

Chapter 59
Case 59: Infusion of Cold Blood. Should We Worry?

A 2½-year-old boy is admitted to a university hospital for wound debridement, dressing change, and skin graft. Two weeks earlier, he had sustained a 14 % total body surface burn. At the other hospital, the child had undergone several uneventful general anesthetics for wound dressing. He is otherwise healthy and the physical exam reveals no abnormalities. His hematocrit (Hct) is 22 % and his platelets count is normal.

A routine general anesthetic ensues and an intravenous (IV) line is inserted in the back of the left hand. The oxygen saturation monitor is on the left index finger, and the blood pressure (BP) cuff is placed on the right arm. The operating room temperature is set at 40 °C. Since the preoperative Hct was low, one unit of warmed packed red blood cells is transfused via gravity. After transfusion, the esophageal temperature increases from 37.1 °C to 39.6 °C. The vital signs are HR 180 beats per minute (bpm), BP 85/35 mmHg, and oxygen saturation 100 %. An arterial blood gas shows a pH 7.47, CO_2 34, oxygen 162, and Hct of 24 %. The blood loss at the time is 300 ml and a new unit of packed cells is given. The unit is not warmed as the child is febrile. The blood is given relatively fast, by manually pressurizing the blood giving set intermittently.

Suddenly, during transfusion, there is a rapid decrease of oxygen saturation from 100 % to 60 %. The pulse tracing is very good and unchanged. You increase the inspired oxygen to 100 %. You stop the pumping of the blood and listen to the chest. You confirm bilateral air entry and hear no adventitious sounds. His mucosa looks pink and the oxygen saturation comes back to 100 %. You pump the blood again and to your dismay the oxygen saturation falls to 40 %.

As a good anesthesiologist you examine the patient. The fingers of the left hand appear dark blue. While the fingers on the right hand are pink. A new oxygen saturation probe on the right hand shows an oxygen saturation of 100 % while the left has an oxygen saturation of 50 %. The latter is shown to increase slowly to 100 %. You have stopped pumping blood and wonder what is going on?

J.G. Brock-Utne, *Near Misses in Pediatric Anesthesia*,   179
DOI 10.1007/978-1-4614-7040-3_59, © Springer Science+Business Media New York 2013

Question

What do you think the problem is?

Solution

Raynaud's phenomenon.

Discussion

Raynaud's phenomenon has been known to be triggered by rapid transfusion of cold blood [1]. In that case, the blood was simply allowed to drip in slowly and no further desaturation occurred. The rest of the anesthetic was uneventful. A small portion of the transfused blood was sent to the blood bank to be tested for possible transfusion reaction. This was negative. Later the child's mother informed the anesthesiologist that during cold weather, the child's fingertips did reversibly turn blue.

In the case above, it was just fortuitous that the IV was on the same hand as the oxygen saturation. If the IV was placed on the other hand, this problem could have remained undiagnosed. A prolonged period of vasoconstriction can cause a potential temporary or permanent injury.

Raynaud's phenomenon has also been reported in adults during blood transfusion [2].

Infusion of cold blood has been known to produce marked prolongation of S-T segments, QRS complex distortion, peaked T-waves, premature ventricular contractions, ventricular fibrillation, and finally bradycardia followed by cardiac arrest [3–5].

Recommendations

1. Raynaud's phenomenon should be suspected when a sudden desaturation occurs when blood is transfused into the same extremity as the oxygen saturation monitor.
2. Blood should always be warmed when given rapidly. Other means of cooling the patient should be used.
3. Having both arms out during a surgical procedure has many advantages including being able to check color, pulses, confirm working of IV, etc.

References

1. Zhang X, Cote CJ. Raynauds's phenomenon in a child presenting as oxygen saturation during transfusion with cold blood. Pediatr Anesth. 2008;18:1208–10.
2. Moore JK, Proctor DW. Raynaud's phenomenon precipitated by blood transfusion. Anaesthesia. 1986;41:398–400.
3. McLean LD, canTyn A. Ventricular defibrillation. JAMA. 1961;175:471.
4. Zauder HL, Yasu O, Orkin LH. Cardiac arrest following massive transfusion. NY State J Med. 1962;62:2400.
5. Boyan CP. Cold or warmed blood for massive transfusions. Ann Surg. 1964;160:282–6.

Chapter 60
Case 60: Respiratory Arrest After Extubation

It is late in the evening. You are taking over a case from one of your colleagues. The patient is an American Society of Anesthesiologists physical status I (ASA 1), 14-year-old girl, 52 kg, and 5′5″. She is having an operation for nonunion of a fractured tibia. The patient is supine and the head is beside the anesthesia machine. Your colleague gives you a full report. You note gas flows, the anesthetic record, and the vital signs. The oxygen tank is full and the pipeline pressure is normal. The suction is attached and working. The patient is otherwise healthy and she has no allergies. There has been minimal blood loss, due to the use of a tourniquet. She is intubated with a #7 endotracheal tube (ETT) and mechanically ventilated. You note no Guedel airway in her mouth, but an esophageal stethoscope with a temperature sensor (DeRoyal, 200 DeBusk Lane, Powell. TN 37849).

Twenty minutes before the surgery ends, you let the patient resume spontaneous breathing and turn the sevoflurane off. Reversal is given and meperidine is titrated to a respiratory rate between 8 and 12 breaths per minute. She is now breathing on N_2O (70 %) in oxygen. The postoperative X-ray of the tibia, done on the operating table, is to the surgeon's satisfaction. He informs you that you can wake up the patient. The N_2O is turned off, the esophageal stethoscope and temperature sensor are removed and the patient awakens. She follows commands and can lift her head. You suck "blindly" in her mouth with a Yankauer suction. A minimal amount of secretion from her oral pharynx is seen. You remove the ETT using the "artificial cough maneuver" [1]. In this maneuver, you close the pop-off valve. When the reservoir bag is distended, you squeeze it, let the ETT cuff down, and quickly remove the ETT, all at the same time. The forced expiration that results with this technique should expel secretions and/or blood around the vocal cords, hence the name. This technique reduces vocal irritation and laryngospasm [1, 2]. However, in this case, after the patient has made a big cough, she attempts to take a big breath but cannot do it. Unable to inhale, she quickly turns cyanotic with tachycardia and hypertension.

J.G. Brock-Utne, *Near Misses in Pediatric Anesthesia*,
DOI 10.1007/978-1-4614-7040-3_60, © Springer Science+Business Media New York 2013

Question

What will you do and what can the problem be?

Solution

A quick look with the laryngoscopy discovers a soft bite block obstructing the laryngeal inlet. The bite block was correctly placed by the initial anesthesiologist. But as mentioned, it had fallen back into the pharynx and was therefore out of view when you removed the tube. It did not help that, when you suctioned the pharynx, you inadvertently pushed the bite block further down.

Discussion

The use of gauze rolls, as soft bite blocks have many supporters. However, soft blocks have several potential problems. Among these are airway obstruction at extubation [3] and the accidental passing of the bite block into the stomach [4].

A potential solution to the problem of dislodgement/misplacement is to make a soft bite block from vaginal packing (either 1″ × 12 ft or 2″ × 15 ft) (National Hospital Packaging, 710 Stimson Avenue, City of Industry, CA 912745). The packing is latex free and is X-ray detectable. The bite block, resembling a cigar, can be made to any size leaving a tail of the packing outside the mouth (Fig. 60.1). The tail can hang free outside the mouth or it can then be secured by tying it to the endotracheal tube (ETT) or attached to a hemostat [5].

A harder bite block can be made from one 4 × 4 gauze, rolled again to look like a cigar, with the use of a rubber tourniquet.[1] The end of the tourniquet can be secured, either to the ETT or to a hemostat.

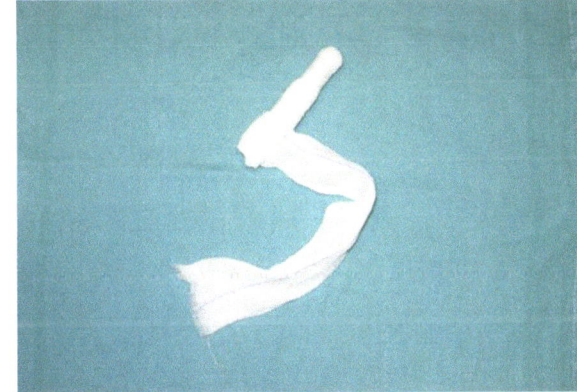

Fig. 60.1 A soft bite block is made from vaginal packing to any size that is needed. The tail that is attached to the bite block can be left outside the mouth. Reproduced courtesy of Brock-Utne and Jaffe [5].

---

[1]Dr. Richard Jaffe personal communication 2012.

Recommendation

Soft bite blocks have many supporters. However, dislodgement/misplacement can occur. Prevention of these problems can be minimized by adding a tail to the soft bite block.

References

1. Landsman IS. Mechanism and treatment of laryngospasm. Int Anesthesiol Clin. 1997;3:67–73.
2. Alamlani A, Ayoub CK, Baraka AS. Laryngospasm: review of different prevention and treatment modalities. (Review article). Pediatr Anesth. 2008;18:281–8.
3. Hasani A. Bite blocks for use in pediatric anesthesia. Pediatr Anesth. 2008;18:1258–9.
4. Khanna P, Pandia MP. Use of bite blocks for pediatric anesthesia. Pediatr Anesth. 2009;19:637.
5. Brock-Utne JG, Jaffe RA. A safety suggestion for soft bite blocks. Pediatr Anesth. 2012;22:1145.

Chapter 61
Case 61: Sudden Increase in End-Tidal CO$_2$

Today your first case of the day is a 2-year-old boy (15 Kg and American Society of Anesthesiologists physical status I [ASA 1]) for an inguinal hernia repair. This is to be his first general anesthetic. His biological parents have not had a general anesthetic, and there is no family history of anesthetic complications.

After being adequately sedated, he is taken to the operating room where the vital signs are HR 112 beats per minute (bpm) sinus rhythm, blood pressure (BP) 85/35, and respiratory rate is 20 breaths per minute. He is given a routine mask induction with sevoflurane in 100 % oxygen, an intravenous (IV) line is placed, and the airway is secured with an endotracheal tube (ETT). Maintenance of anesthesia is with fentanyl, rocuronium, sevoflurane (2 %) in 70 % nitrous oxide in oxygen. The fresh gas flow is 1.5 min. An upper body Bair Hugger (Augustine medical Inc. Eden Prairie, MN) is placed and a heat moisture exchanger (HME) (Kimberley Clark Ballard 1000) is inserted between the ETT and the Y-piece of the circle system. The patient is ventilated with a peak inspiratory pressure of 17 cm and a tidal volume of 95 ml. His vital signs are HR 100, BP 80/40, esophageal temperature 36.5 °C, and end-tidal carbon dioxide (CO$_2$) 32 mmHg.

Thirty-five minutes into the case, the end-tidal CO$_2$ increases rapidly to 52 mmHg and the HR goes to 128 bpm. The temperature is 36.2 °C. The peak airway pressure remains at 17 cm H$_2$O. Examination of the chest shows bilateral air entry with no adventitious sounds. His pupils are constricted and you consider him adequately anesthetized. The CO$_2$ absorber is only slightly discolored, meaning that your soda lime is not exhausted. You increased the fresh gas flow to 4 l/min, tidal volume to 110 ml, and the ventilator rate to 22 bpm, but there are only slight decreases in both end-tidal CO$_2$ and heart rate.

Question

What is the first thing to do, to try to normalize the end-tidal CO$_2$ and heart rate and what would you include in your list of differential diagnoses?

Solution

Remove the HME.

In a previous case [1], there was a prompt normalization of both abnormal parameters within <3 min after the removal of the HME.

Discussion

The differential diagnoses included faulty expiratory valve, thyroid storm, hypoventilation, increased dead space, light anesthesia, exhausted soda lime, and a malfunctioning CO_2 absorber.

The fact that the end-tidal CO_2 and the heart rate improved so quickly after removal of the HME can only be attributed to an increased dead space within the HME [2, 3]. The tachycardia was thought to be due to respiratory acidosis, which stimulated the sympathetic nervous system [1].

It is interesting that in this case [1] there was no associated increase in inspiratory and expiratory resistance. Also in this case, the administration of the HME to the circuit increased the dead space by nearly 70 % [1]. For more information about the anatomic dead space in infants, see the paper by Numa and Newth [4].

Recommendation

HMEs in pediatric anesthesia can cause hypoventilation and tachycardia during intermittent positive-pressure ventilation (IPPV).

References

1. Karlin A, Umeh U, Girshin M. Hypercapnia and tachycardia in a 2-year-old. Pediatr Anesth. 2009;19:629–30.
2. Campbell RS, David Jr K, Johannigman JA, Branson RD. The effects of passive humidifier dead space on respiratory variables in paralyzed and spontaneously breathing patients. Respir Care. 2000;45:306–12.
3. Johnson PA, Raper RF, Fisher MM. The impact of heat and moisture exchanging humidifiers on work of breathing. Anaesth Intensive Care. 1995;23:697–701.
4. Numa AH, Newth CJ. Anatomic dead space in infants and children. J Appl Physiol. 1996;80:1485–9.

Chapter 62
Case 62: A Case of Acute Lymphoblastic Leukemia (ALL)

A 5-year-old boy (20 kg) with a diagnosis of acute lymphoblastic leukemia (ALL) is scheduled for a lumbar puncture with intrathecal injection of methotrexate and placement of a Port-a-Cath. The boy was diagnosed with ALL 4 weeks before. At that time, a chemotherapy regimen was commenced (vincristine, dexamethasone, and asparaginase). Previous anesthetic before the diagnosis of ALL had been uneventful. His preoperative hematology and clotting studies were normal. Electrolyte panel was not done.

After a midazolam premedication, he is taken to the operating room. An intravenous line (IV) is placed and you induce him with 20 mcg of fentanyl and propofol 100 mg. After this dose, the child does not seem to be "asleep" and you give another dose of propofol 50 mg and another 50 mg. A total of 200 mg is now given over a 2–4-min period. His vital signs remain stable and he is easy to mask ventilate. A non-depolarizing muscle relaxation (atracurium 10 mg) is given and the trachea intubated with an endotracheal tube #5. Positive pressure ventilation ensues and bilateral air entry is heard. The anesthetic is maintained with 50–50 mixtures of air and oxygen and isoflurane. You note that the inspired isoflurane concentration is 2.5 % while the end-tidal isoflurane concentration has only reached 0.75 %. You recheck the anesthesia machine. You find no leaks or other concerns. Peak pressures remain the same and there is bilateral air entry. Just to be sure a second anesthesia gas monitor is brought in, but the same differences between the inspired and end-tidal isoflurane concentrations are seen. Since the patient appears "light" (moving in response to surgical stimulus), you increase the inspired isoflurane concentration to >4 %. With this concentration, you see end-tidal isoflurane concentrations rise to 1.2 1.5 %. However, the patient remains somewhat reactive to surgical stimulus despite no twitches with a total of 3 mcg/kg of fentanyl.

At the end of the procedure, which lasted 75 min, the patient is reversed and spontaneous breathing resumes. He is, however, slow to awaken. It is then that the surgeon comments that he thought the blood looked very "milky." You dismiss the comment as you do not know what that has to do with a slow wake up. The patient is taken to the recovery room where he slowly wakes up over a 30-min period. The rest of his postoperative course is uneventful.

J.G. Brock-Utne, *Near Misses in Pediatric Anesthesia*, 191
DOI 10.1007/978-1-4614-7040-3_62, © Springer Science+Business Media New York 2013

Your second child (American Society of Anesthesiologists physical status I [ASA 1]) in the same room with the same machine and anesthetic technique is totally uneventful. In this case, the inspired and expired isoflurane concentrations are similar.

Question

You are at a loss to understand what the problem could have been with the first case. Do you have any idea?

Solution

In a case, like the one previously cited, Moore and Smith [1] from Great Ormond Street Hospital, London, UK, suggested that the problem was due to preexisting severe hyperlipidemia.

Discussion

In their case [1], the preoperative blood results showed significant hyperlipidemia. The cholesterol was 11.7 mmol/L (Normal range 2.8–4.8 mmol/L.) and his triglyceride was 14.4 mmol/L (Normal range 0.36–4.8 mmol/L). The current treatment of ALL including dexamethsone and asparaginase causes transient hyperlipidemia [2, 3]. Asparaginase is suggested to affect lipid metabolism by increasing synthesis of VLDL (very low density lipoprotein) and inhibiting lipoprotein lipase activity. The latter will increase plasma triglycerides. Moore and Smith [1] suggest that the patient's severe hyperlipidemia significantly increased the solubility of isoflurane in the blood. This leads to a wide difference in inspired and end-tidal isoflurane concentrations. This could therefore explain the slow onset of anesthesia and a delay in recovery.

Fentanyl action can also have been affected by hyperlipidemia as it is also relatively lipid soluble [4]. Hyperlipidemia will therefore act rather as a reservoir for fentanyl [4].

Note that hyperlipidemia can also effect the measurement of electrolytes and urea [5].

Recommendation

This case highlights the possibility that hyperlipidemia could potentially cause a slow onset of anesthesia and a delay in recovery.

References

1. Moore J, Smith JII. A case of resistance to anesthesia secondary to severe hyperlipidemia. Pediatr Anesth. 2007;17:1223–4.
2. Steinherz PG. Transient and severe hyperlipidemia in patients with acute lymphoblastic leukemia treated with prednisone and asparaginase. Cancer. 1994;74:3234–9.
3. Tozuka M, Yamauchi K, Hidaka H, Nakabayashi T, Okumura N, Katsuyama T. Characterization of hypertriglyceridemia induced by L-asparaginase therapy for acute lymphoblastic leukemia and malignant lymphoma. Ann Clin Lab Sci. 1997;27:351–7.
4. Wasan KM. Modifications in plasma lipoprotein concentration and lipid composition regulate the biological activity of hydrophobic drugs. J Pharmacol Toxicol Methods. 1996;36:1–11.
5. Kroll MH, Elin RJ. Interference with clinical laboratory analysis. Clin Chem. 1994;40:1996–2005.

Chapter 63
Case 63: Intraoperative Airway Obstruction

A 22-month-old (15 kg) boy is scheduled for an orthopedic procedure on his right foot in a prone position. The boy is otherwise healthy with normal milestones. This is his first operation. His family history is negative for anesthesia complications.

After adequate sedation, he is taken to the operating room. Routine American Society of Anesthesiologists (ASA) monitors are placed. A mask induction with sevoflurane and nitrous oxide in oxygen is uneventful. An intravenous (IV) line is placed in his left hand and his trachea intubated with an endotracheal tube 4.0 (ETT) under propofol sedation. Bilateral air entry is heard and normal end tidal carbon dioxide (ETCO$_2$) waveforms are noted. The child's head is lying on a foam pad. Before turning the patient prone you make a passage, with a scissors, for the ETT in the foam face pad. From previous experience, you have found this useful when the patient is in the prone position. The patient is disconnected from the anesthesia circuit and positioned prone. His face is placed in the foam pad above and the anesthesia circuit reconnected. However, you see that the peak pressure is now dramatically increased and the tidal volume and ETCO$_2$ go to zero. You confirm high peak pressures by attempting to ventilate manually. There is no kink in the ETT. You pass an 8F soft suction catheter, but it stops halfway down the ETT. You suspect a foreign body in the ETT and quickly turn the child over, remove the offending ETT, and reintubate with a new one. The vital signs return to normal and the patient is again placed in the prone position. The operation is concluded uneventfully.

Question

You inspect the ETT that has been removed and discover a foreign body lodged inside it. What can the foreign body be?

J.G. Brock-Utne, *Near Misses in Pediatric Anesthesia*,
DOI 10.1007/978-1-4614-7040-3_63, © Springer Science+Business Media New York 2013

Solution

In a previous case, the foreign body was a 12×4×5 mm piece of foam [1]. This foam piece could only have come from the face pad that had been cut.

Discussion

In the case above [1], the authors elected to use a 10F soft suction catheter after using the 8F catheter. With the 10F, they were able to suck the piece of foam from the ETT without turning the patient supine. Throughout their management, the oxygen saturation was above 96 % and the heart rate never went below 100 beats per minute (bpm). After the foam was removed from the ETT, the case proceeded uneventfully.

Personally, I would have dealt with this problem the way I outlined on the previous page. What would they have done if the use of the 10F suction catheter had been unsuccessful? They would then have to turn the child supine, remove the ETT, and reintubate. But as we know, all that takes time.

The other danger in a case like this one is the positive pressure ventilation could have pushed the foam into the bronchial tree and cause a serious life-threatening complication. This may have occurred if you had not diagnosed the foreign body, but thought the patient had a bronchospasm and ventilated with albuterol.

Recommendation

Foam face pads have proved to be safe and effective. However, if you elect to modify the pad with a scalpel or a scissors, be aware that small pieces of foam may become dislodged and enter into your patient's ETT.

Reference

1. Walker BJ, Rampersad SE. Iatrogenic endotracheal tube obstruction with foam face padding. Pediatr Anesth. 2009;19:544–5.

Chapter 64
Case 64: An Anterior Mediastinal Mass. What Will You Do?

An 18-year-old boy is an "add on" in a large university hospital. It is 6 p.m. He is scheduled for a thoracoscopy and biopsy. He has recently been diagnosed with a 13 cm anterior mediastinal mass. The mass on computed tomography scan shows the arch vessels, superior vena cava, and trachea all encasing these structures. The distal trachea and the right main bronchus are 60 % compressed. You go and see the patient. He is surrounded by his family who are all very concerned. The surgeon is also at the bedside. He introduces you by saying, "This anesthesiologist will make sure that you get a safe general anesthetic."

The young man (55 Kg) denies dyspnea, orthopnea, or coughing when lying down. You examine in his neck and discover a few small and one big cervical lymph gland. There are decreased breath sounds of the right apical lung field. The breath sounds are normal and there is no evidence of stridor. His vital signs, including the oxygen saturation on room air (97), are within normal limits.

Question

As mentioned, it is late in the day and the surgeon is keen to get going ASAP. How would you proceed?

Solution

Suggest to the surgeon that the cervical lymph glands should be removed under local anesthesia.

Discussion

A similar case [1] has been described. In that case, general anesthesia was induced with an inhalation technique using sevoflurane (8 %) in 100 % oxygen. The patient was left breathing spontaneously through an endotracheal tube (ETT). No muscle relaxants were used when placing the ETT. While the surgeon performed bronchoscopy and the patient was breathing spontaneously, the oxygen saturation and end-tidal CO_2 fell precipitously. On examination, it was noted that the air entry into the entire right lung was decreased. The bronchoscope was removed and the surgical team prepared for an emergency cardiopulmonary bypass (CPB). The anesthetic gas was turned off and various maneuvers were instituted to improve oxygenation. As the patient began to wake up, the vital signs improved and air entry was again heard in the patient's right lung field. The patient made an uneventful recovery. Next day, the cervical lymph nodes were biopsied under local anesthesia.

Airway and vascular collapse are well-known complications in patients with an anterior mediastinal mass [2]. Other anesthetic problems in these cases include difficulty in extubation and/or diminished lung volumes [3]. It is recommended that local anesthesia is used in these cases when there is an accessible cervical lymph node [2–4].

Unfortunately, there are cases where there are no extrathoracic lymph nodes, and in these cases, general anesthesia must be induced. As a precaution, one should always have a rigid bronchoscope available (however in this case it seemed to have initiated the problem). Also it is essential to have the option to place the patient rapidly on CPB.

One case report has reported no adverse events in the perioperative period when using dexmedetomidine and ketamine for a large anterior mediastinal mass biopsy in a 4-year-old [5]. It is interesting to note that ketamine is not associated with loss of airway patency or with a decrease in airway muscle activity. On the other hand, midazolam is associated with a significant decrease in muscle activity with an increase in airway obstruction [6]. Dexmedetomidine's effect on airway muscle tone is unknown [5].

Recommendation

Remember we as anesthesiologists are physicians, not technicians to do what we are told. Always examine your patient. In this case, a discussion with the patient, the family, and the surgeon about doing this case under local anesthesia would have been not only correct, but potentially lifesaving. Also, take into account that in this age group, an anterior mediastinal mass is most likely a curable disease. To submit the child to a near lethal procedure by administrating a general anesthetic is obviously not good care.

References

1. Gardner JC, Royster RL. Airway collapse with an anterior mediastinal mass despite spontaneous ventilation in an adult. Anesth Analg. 2011;113:239–42.
2. Blank RS, de Souza DG. Anesthetic management of patients with an anterior mediastinal mass: continuing professional development. Can J Anesth. 2011;58:853–67.
3. Gothard JWW. Anesthetic consideration for patients with anterior mediastinal masses. Anesthesiol Clin. 2008;26:305–14.
4. Thompson A. Anterior mediastinal masses: Look before you leap. Anesth Analg. 2012;114:476.
5. Mahmoud M, Tyler T, Sadhasivam S. Dexmedetomidine and ketamine for large anterior mediastinal mass biopsy. Pediatr Anesth. 2008;18:976–1014.
6. Drummond GB. Comparison of sedation with midazolam and ketamine: effects on airway muscle activity. Br J Anaesth. 1996;76:663–7.

Chapter 65
Case 65: A "Routine" MRI Case

Today you are scheduled to work with a Certified Registered Nurse Anesthetist (CRNA) in the magnetic resonance imaging (MRI) suite. The patient is a 17-year-old boy (72 kg). He was diagnosed 3 weeks ago with acute transverse myelitis. He presented with acute and progressive bilateral leg weakness and bladder dysfunction. Since he suffered from severe claustrophobia, he underwent an MRI of his spine and head under propofol infusion. The propofol recovery was very delayed due to excessive somnolence. His vital signs remained stable. Otherwise, the procedure was uneventful. He was started on intravenous (IV) steroids and IV immunoglobulin. Now 3 weeks after the onset, he is showing signs of neurological recovery. A repeat MRI is requested.

You see and examine the boy in the preoperative area. He is alert and orientated for time and place. His vital signs are normal. On physical exam, you note 3/5 weakness of his lower limbs. There is no paraesthesia. The CRNA suggests dexmedetomidine as the sole anesthetic/sedative agent, because of the previous slow recovery with propofol.

Question

You agree that this seems like a good idea, but is it?

J.G. Brock-Utne, *Near Misses in Pediatric Anesthesia*,
DOI 10.1007/978-1-4614-7040-3_65, © Springer Science+Business Media New York 2013

Solution

It may not be, as a previously similar case report [1] reported severe hypertension and bradycardia within 8 min of infusing dexmedetomidine.

Discussion

In the previous report [1], a loading dose of 2 mcg/kg of dexmedetomidine led to severe hypertension (230/120) and bradycardia (dropping from 70 to low 30s). The dexmedetomidine was stopped and the MRI was completed successfully with propofol infusion.

Acute transverse myelitis is a focal inflammatory disease of the spinal cord. It results in motor, sensory, and autonomic dysfunction [2]. The authors [1] theorized that the cause of their patient's hypertension and bradycardia was the patient's lack of inhibiter spinal reflexes. Without the inhibitory reflexes, dexmedetomdine led to an exaggerated response causing peripheral vasoconstriction.

In healthy adult volunteers, a biphasic effect following dexmedetomidine is usually seen [1]. Initially there is an increase, lasting 5–10 min, in systolic blood pressure (SBP) and reflex bradycardia. The reason for this change is that the drug initially stimulates the peripheral postsynaptic (alpha) 2B adrenergic receptor, causing peripheral vasoconstriction with the resultant increase in SBP. Eventually, after 5–10 min, the drug decreases SBP and normalizes the heart rate as a result of central presynaptic (alpha) 2A adrenergic receptor's stimulation [3].

Recommendation

One of my early teachers of anesthesia (Jon Gjessing, 1971, Sundsvall, Sweden) always said, "A sedated patient in the recovery room is a good thing. That it lasts a little longer than normal, when everything else is normal, is still a good thing. Don't worry about it."

He also said, "In the same patient never change a previously winning anesthetic technique."

We will never know what would have happened if the second MRI had been done with propofol initially, but we do know that propofol was successful in the second MRI, when dexmedetomidine was not.

References

1. Shah S, Sangai T, Quasim M, Martin T. Severe hypertension and bradycardia with dexmedetomidine for radiology sedation in a patient with acute transverse myelitis. Pediatr Anesth. 2008;18:667–92.
2. Transverse Myelitis consortium working group. Proposed diagnostic criteria and nosology of acute transverse myelitis. Neurology. 2002;59:499–505.
3. Hall JE, Uhrich TD, Barney JA, Arain SR, Ebert TJ. Sedative, amnestic and analgesic properties of small-dose dexmedetomidine infusions. Anesth Analg. 2000;90:699–705.

Chapter 66
Case 66: A Serious Problem During Neurosurgery

It is late in the evening and you are taking over the anesthetic management of a patient from one of your colleagues. The case is a 6-year-old female (American Society of Anesthesiologists physical status II [ASA 2], 15 kg) who has been undergoing a 3 h craniotomy in the prone position for a cerebellar tumor. The child is turned 180° away from you. There are no other medical or surgical issues with the patient. She has been started on Tegretol for seizures.

Your colleague gives you a report. The last dose of rocuronium was at induction. There has been minimal blood loss. The vital signs are normal. You crawl under the operating table and with your gloved hands feel that the endotracheal tube (ETT) is secure and the eyes are not being pressurized. It is impossible to verify anything by sight. As you crawl back to the anesthesia machine, you notice that there is blood on your gloved fingers from having touched the ETT. You presume that the blood must be from the operating site.

Your colleague leaves and you settle down to do your charting. Suddenly you notice that there is a neurologist in the room, something that your colleague forgot to mention. The neurologist tells you that he has been doing motor-evoked potential monitoring (MEPM) for the last several hours. You now understand why no more rocuronium was given.

Question

Should you be concerned and what will you do?

Solution

Check what type of bite block has been used and if it is still there.

Discussion

This happened to a friend of mine. When he went under the operating table again to investigate what sort of bite block was used, he found none. A soft block was seen on the floor. He inserted a BiteGard (Hudson RCI, Teleflex Medical, Research Triangle Park, NC 27709, USA) between the molars. In Stanford, we have used the BiteGard for more than 4 years with no adverse events. The BiteGard has a handle attached to the teeth guard. The handle protrudes from the mouth and can be secured to the ETT, teeth, or face with tape or silk. At the end of the above case, fortunately, the damage to the tongue was slight and no further treatment was needed.

In anesthetized/sedated intubated patients, it is necessary to maintain the lumen of the ETT. Biting on the tube may obstruct, damage, or cut the ETT in half. The use of a strong bite block or an oropharyngeal (Guedel) airway should be employed to keep the ETT lumen patent [1]. However, it has been reported that the Guedel airway is not without problems. These include edema of lips and tongue, bleeding, hoarseness, and sore throat [2–4]. However, of more concern is the article by Monroe et al. [5] that states that the Guedel airway may compress the base of the tongue, resulting in ischemia and venous congestion, causing macroglossia and ischemic necrosis of the tongue. I have seen macroglossia but no ischemia of the tongue. The correct size of the Guedel is the key in the prevention of ischemia from happening.

It is imperative that a soft bite block is not used in any case where motor-evoked potential monitoring (MEPM) will be used. A soft bite block will not prevent trauma to teeth or tongue or lips [6]. Furthermore, the block that is employed must not fall out or move during general anesthesia. This is especially true when MEPM is being used. Should the tongue or lips get between the teeth instead of the bite block, severe tongue laceration can occur [7]. This is due to repetitive jaw muscle contractions during MEPM.

No more is this a problem when the patient is prone, as the bite block may fall out and the tongue protrudes out of the mouth.

Lastly, the protruding handle of the BiteGard block reminds the physician that it has been used and must be removed intact prior to extubation.

Recommendation

A soft bite block should not be used in cases where MEPM is being employed in neurosurgery or spine cases. Commercially available bite blocks should be employed in these cases and secured (so they do not fall out) when the patient is in the prone position [8].

References

1. Baskett T. Arthur Guedel and the oropharyngeal airway. Resuscitation. 2004;63:3–5.
2. Pivalizza EG, Katz J, Singh S, Liu W, McGraw-Wall BL. Massive macroglossia after posterior fossa surgery in the prone position. J Neurosurg Anesthesiol. 1998;10:34–6.
3. Kuhnert SM, Faust RJ, Berge KH, Piepgras DG. Postoperative macroglossia: report of a case with rapid resolution after extubation of the trachea. Anesth Analg. 1999;88:220–3.
4. Drummond JC, Kuhnert SM, Piepgras DG. Macroglossia. Déjà vu Response. Anesth Analg. 1999;89:534.
5. Monroe MC, Gravenstein N, Saga-Rumley S. Postoperative sore throat; effect of oropharyngeal airway in orotracheally intubated patients. Anesth Analg. 1990;70:512–6.
6. Deiner SG, Osborn IP. Prevention of airway injury during spine surgery: rethinking bite blocks. J Neurosurg Anesthesiol. 2009;21:68–9.
7. Tamkus A, Rice K. The incidence of bite injuries associated with the transcranial motor-evoked potential monitoring. Anesth Analg. 2012;115(3):663–7. Epub 2012 Apr 20.
8. Brock-Utne JG, Jaffe RA. Motor-evoked potential monitoring and the prone patient. Pediatr Anesth. 2013;22:205–207.

Chapter 67
Case 67: A Case of Severe Intra-abdominal Pressure

You are on a mission trip to an underdeveloped country providing anesthesia to elective cleft lip repair. You have just arrived and it is late at night. The local hospital surgeon finds you and wonders if you could come and help with an emergency. He is unable to find the anesthesiologist on call.

The case is a 3-year-old boy (14 kg) who was an unrestrained passenger in a motor vehicle accident (MVA). It is reported that the MVA happened more than 48 h ago. But it is more likely to be at least 3 days ago, as the accident happened in a remote part of the country and far away from this hospital.

The surgeon carries the child into the operating room (OR) as you are getting ready. He places the child on the OR table. The boy's Glasgow coma scale is 11/15. His vital signs are as follows: the heart rate (HR) 140 beats per minute (bpm), respiration 40/min, blood pressure (BP) 80/60 mmHg, and the oxygen saturation is 80–84 % on room air. A very distended and tender abdomen is felt. On percussion, it does not sound like air. With a flashlight (shining through the abdomen from the lateral side) you establish that it looks like fluid, most likely urine. You diagnose a ruptured bladder. The surgeon concurs. The child is breathing spontaneously, but labored, via an oxygen face mask. Examination of heart and lung is normal, except air entry is poor in the lower and middle lung fields, both anterior and posterior. Preoxygenation only brings the oxygen saturation to 92 %.

You do a rapid sequence induction with ketamine and succinylcholine. Cricoid pressure is maintained and the endotracheal tube (ETT) is rapidly passed into the trachea. The cuff is inflated. Unfortunately it is virtually impossible to manually ventilate the child, as the airway pressures are over 70 cm H_2O. You confirm that the ETT is patent with a suction catheter and that the tube is in the correct place, as anteriorly you hear distant breath sounds bilaterally. The oxygen saturation declines further and very little end-tidal CO_2 is seen. The HR is now falling to 70 bpm.

J.G. Brock-Utne, *Near Misses in Pediatric Anesthesia*,
DOI 10.1007/978-1-4614-7040-3_67, © Springer Science+Business Media New York 2013

Question

What will you do?

Solution

Ask the surgeon, without waiting for proper prep and drape, to make an incision in the lower abdomen to release the pressure caused by the urine.

Discussion

This case is similar to a case described [1]. After the lower abdominal incision was made, a large amount of fluid shot out. Ventilation improved with a suction placed in the abdominal cavity. Oxygen saturation increased to 99 % and end tidal CO_2 increased and returned to normal within minutes. The fluid collected in the case [1] was 2.3 l consisting mainly of urine. The bladder was repaired and the child made an uneventful recovery.

With muscle paralysis, the muscle tone of the diaphragm disappears. The intra-abdominal volume, in this case mainly urine, pushed the diaphragm cephalad. To attempt to ventilate against this resistance, the peak airway pressures increased dramatically resulting in decreased tidal volume, oxygen saturation, venous return, and cardiac output.

It is more common to encounter blood in the peritoneal cavity than urine. This can occur following a trauma or an ectopic pregnancy. In these cases, as the intra-abdominal pressure increases, it often prevents exsanguination. The increased free blood in the peritoneal cavity acts as a "pressure bandage." After an anesthetic induction the BP may drop, but more usually it falls precipitously after the surgeon has made his/her incision. In these cases, it is imperative that you have blood in the room and at least two working large bore IVs.

I have seen a similar case (ASA 4E—American Society of Anesthesiologists physical status IV emergency) in which the abdomen was so distended by a ruptured bowel from typhoid. After induction, it became nearly impossible to ventilate. Dr. Bob Mickel (Professor of Pediatric Surgery, University of Natal, Durban, South Africa), a wonderful and gifted pediatric surgeon, saved the child by rapidly making a surgical incision and releasing both gas and fluid. The child survived the operation, only to die a few days later of the disease.

As mentioned in Case 1 of this book, excessive air insufflation during gastrointestinal endoscopy can also increase peak airway pressures, leading to oxygen desaturation, etc. [2].

Recommendation

When faced with a massive increase in peak airway pressure, caused by excessive intra-abdominal fluid, it is imperative to have a competent surgeon in the room.

References

1. Ghaffari S. Difficult ventilation from increased abdominal pressure. Pediatr Anesth. 2007;17:187–8.
2. Brock-Utne JG, Moynihan RJ. Patient draping contributing to the near disaster (desaturation during endoscopy in a 2-year-old). Pediatr Anesth. 1992;2:333–4.

Chapter 68
Case 68: A Case of Severe Laryngospasm

A 4-year-old girl (American Society of Anesthesiologists physical status I [ASA 1], 20 kg) is scheduled for elective tonsillectomy. She is otherwise healthy. There is no family history of anesthetic mishaps or concerns. Four weeks before, she had an upper respiratory tract infection.

You see her in the preoperative area. On exam her chest is clear and enlarged tonsils are seen, but they are not inflamed. She has been fasting for 6 h. She is taken to the operating room (OR) having been adequately sedated with oral midazolam. Her vital signs are normal, heart rate (HR) 105 beats per minute (bpm), blood pressure (BP) 80/50, and oxygen saturation is 99 % on room air.

Routine inhalational induction with sevoflurane ensues and an intravenous (IV) line is placed. The patient is paralyzed and manually ventilated with a mask. A grade 1 view is seen on laryngoscopy and endotracheal intubation is accomplished. End-tidal CO_2 is seen and bilateral air entry is heard. The surgery is completed within 1 h and the sevoflurane is turned off. Reversal is given and spontaneous ventilation resumes in nitrous oxide 50 % in oxygen. IV meperidine is administered to get a respiratory rate of 8–12 per min. The respiration is seen to be regular and rhythmic. The nitrous oxide is turned off and the child opens her eyes. You remove the endotracheal tube (ETT) with the child in the right lateral position. Immediately there is evidence of airway obstruction with inspiratory stridor and suprasternal retraction. You do your jaw thrust and apply manual positive pressure with 100 % oxygen. Despite these efforts, the oxygen saturation drops from 98 % to 86 % and the HR decreases to 80 bpm. The values are seen to decrease as you look at the monitors. You consider various options for treating laryngospasm, like (1) the gold standard succinylcholine 1–2 mg/kg with atropine 0.02 mg/kg if there is bradycardia or (2) just a smaller dose of succinylcholine (0.1 mg/kg). You dismiss the ideas of a small dose of propofol (0.5–0.8 mg/kg) as its role in breaking a laryngospasm in the presence of bradycardia is not proven to be either safe or effective [1]. Since you do not have any IV nitroglycerine, you dismiss a small dose of this drug (4 µg/kg) [2].

Question

Is there any other maneuver you would suggest before giving your succinylcholine?

Solution

A gentle chest compression that produces exhalation.

Discussion

In my early days of training (1972), an older and wiser man called Geoffrey (Geoff) Barwise (senior consultant, King Edward 8 Hospital, Durban, South Africa) came to my aid in a similar case. Geoff told me to continue with the jaw thrust but to stop for 2–4 s giving positive pressure with the tight-fitting face mask with 100 % oxygen. With no positive pressure, Geoff gently gave a few chest compressions. The results were miraculous. Since then, I have always used this technique with great success. Only twice I have had to resort to succinylcholine.

Recently, in a prospective study of 1,226 children, gentle chest compression with 100 % oxygen via the mask was successful in the immediate management of postextubation laryngeal spasm [3]. It was interesting that none of the children in the chest compression group developed gastric distention, compared to 86.5 % in the non-compression group.

Sometimes in cases of severe laryngospasm, you may lose the airway and also have no IV. Succinylcholine may be indicated. I recommend you read the editorial entitled: "Which port in a storm? Use of suxamethonium without intravenous access for severe laryngospasm" [4]. Despite the fact that there is a reported increased incidence of arrhythmias with the intralingual/submental routes, it has worked successfully for me many times. It is most important to remember that in these cases, a rapid decision to give succinylcholine may save the day. Don't hesitate.

Recommendation

Gentle chest compression (Barwise) with a jaw thrust may prove to be a simple and effective technique for the management of postextubation laryngeal spasm in children. If that does not work, give succinlycholine.

References

1. Hampson-Evans D, Morgan P, Farrar M. Pediatric laryngospasm. Pediatr Anesth. 2008;18:303–7.
2. Alalami AA, Ayoub CM, Baraka AS. Laryngospasm: review of different prevention and treatment modalities. Pediatr Anesth. 2008;18:281–8.
3. Al-Metwallik RR, Mowafi HA, Ismail SA. Gentle chest compression relieves extubation laryngospasm in children. J Anesth. 2010;24:854–7.
4. Walker RWM, Sutton RS. Which port in a storm? Use of suxamethonium without intravenous access for severe laryngospasm. Anaesthesia. 2007;62:757–9.

Chapter 69
Case 69: An ETT Suction Problem

A 5-week-old girl (4 kg) is admitted from a rural hospital via helicopter. She is diagnosed with a lower respiratory tract infection, which, after 2 days in the rural hospital, has now progressed to respiratory failure. You see the child immediately on arrival in the emergency room (ER). The child is struggling and the oxygen saturation has fallen to 84 % in the last few minutes. You quickly place an orally 3.5 endotracheal tube (ETT) and the vital signs improve dramatically. The ETT was cut by you prior to the insertion to get the correct length of the ETT. Prior to the ETT being placed in the trachea, the International Organization for Standardization (ISO) connector is attached to the ETT, however with some difficulty. (See Case 48 for a better way to put the ISO connector on the ETT after the tube has been cut). Two hours later, you get a call from the intensive care unit (ICU) telling you that it is not possible to pass any sized suction catheter down the ETT.

You arrive and find the vital signs are stable but the child requires suctioning. The child is paralyzed, ventilated, and sedated. The nurse tells you that the peak pressures have not changed much.

Question

Like a good anesthesiologist you never trust anyone. You attempt to pass several suction catheters through the ETT but you can only confirm the ICU nurse's findings. The catheter stopped after a very short distance. The tip does not seem to get past the ISO connector. Besides replacing the ETT, is there anything else you could do to make the ETT suction successful?

Solution

If possible, remove the ISO connector and replace it with a new one. If that cannot be done, then replace the ETT. When examining the removed ETT, you will notice that the tip of the ISO connector is indented [1]. The indentation causes the lumen to be narrowed and partially obstructed. The damage to the ISO connector is thought to be caused when the connector is being pushed into the ETT [2]. The latter can be difficult, as the diameter of the ETT, when it is cut, is usually narrower compared to the proximal end of the ETT with the connector.

Discussion

The shortening of the ETT is done to decrease dead space and resistance to flow [3]. It is also done to decrease the likelihood of dislodgment and kinking and to make suctioning easier [1]. Cutting a nasal or an oral ETT after it has been placed in the trachea is common practice. Be aware that the ISO connector can be damaged when inserting it into the cut ETT. The damage is usually in the form of an indentation of the tip of the ISO connector. This can lead to narrowing of the lumen, thereby preventing suction catheters to be inserted. Because of this potential problem, many anesthesiologists cut the ETT to a desired length prior to its use and place the distal end of the ETT in warm water prior to the connector's insertion. Warming the ETT will make the connector slide in easier. Others have reported ETT connector fractures [1, 4] that may have been related to the use of forceps in the reattachment process [4].

Recommendation

An ISO connector can be damaged during reinsertion into an ETT, causing a narrowing of the lumen. This can lead to an inability to suction the ETT with a suction catheter, or worse, an inability to ventilate.

References

1. Guruswamy V, Parkins K. Faulty tracheal tube connector. Anaesthesia. 2006;61:915–6.
2. Johnston S, Holmes P. Potential hazard of endotracheal tube ISO connector. Pediatr Anesth. 2009;19:1247–9.
3. Manczur T, Greenough A, Nicholsan GP, Rafferty GF. Resistance of pediatric and neonatal endotracheal tubes; influences of flow rate, size and shape. Crit Care Med. 2000;28:1595–8.
4. Nixon C. Endotracheal tube connector fracture – an avoidable hazard. Can J Anaesth. 1986;33:251–2.

Chapter 70
Case 70: A Child Refusing an Operation

It is the first case of the day. The patient is a 10-year-old girl (American Society of Anesthesiologists physical status I [ASA 1]) scheduled for repair of prominent ears. The parents, who accompany the child, are very keen to have the ears corrected. The child, on other the hand, is worried and asks if she can go home. She tells you that she is anxious, as she has seen a film that showed a person who was paralyzed and aware during anesthesia. The girl seems intelligent and articulates her concerns very well.

When offered the oral midazolam, she refuses to take it and states clearly, "I want to go home." To which the parents say, "No way." There is a bit of an awkward moment and the girl says, "I don't worry about the ears. I am fine as I am."

To which the mother replies, "But you are teased by the children in the school because they stick out. We are only looking after your best interest. You will be much happier with the ears corrected."

The father nods his head and says, "I have taken time off from work to come here. Be reasonable and let's get this done. You will be much happier."

Question

The surgeon is not taking sides and leaves the bedside. Left with this potential dilemma, what would you do?

J.G. Brock-Utne, *Near Misses in Pediatric Anesthesia*,
DOI 10.1007/978-1-4614-7040-3_70, © Springer Science+Business Media New York 2013

Solution

Postpone the operation, based on the fact that you are unwilling to force the child to undergo an elective operation. Even though the parents have signed the consent, you should take into account the girl's refusal. This is an elective procedure and the child should not be forced to have the ears corrected if she does not want it.

Discussion

All children have a legal and ethical right to have their views heard and considered on matters that could have a bad outcome [1, 2].

It is not an option to take this unpremedicated girl into the operating room and holding her down for a mask induction. Some may have considered placing an intravenous (IV) line and giving midazolam IV to calm her down. I would not recommend that. This is an elective surgery. In these situations, time should be given to allow for further consultation so that you can ensure that the "greatest good" is done with the least possible harm/damage.

On the other hand, if this was a necessary medical/surgical treatment, the child has no right to refuse when harm will be done to the child should medical/surgical treatment not be instituted.

Recommendation

Children have a legal and ethical right to voice their concerns on matters that may affect them in an adverse way.

References

1. Walker H. The child who refuses to undergo anesthesia and surgery – a case scenario-based discussion of the ethical and legal issues. Pediatr Anesth. 2009;19:1017–21.
2. Multitude of authors. Special themed issue on ethics. Pediatr Anesth. 2009;19:931–1021.

Chapter 71
Case 71: Why So Sleepy?

It is late at night. You are on call and taking over a case from one of your colleagues. The case is a correction of scoliosis in a 16-year-old girl. The operation has been going for 8 h. The anesthesiologist gives you a detailed account of the anesthetic, which includes nitrous oxide in oxygen and isoflurane 1–1.5 %. Fortunately it has been uneventful and the blood loss has been only 500 ml. The patient's vital signs are within normal limits. They have about an hour left. You check the anesthesia machine which is a Dräger Apollo anesthesia workstation. You find everything in order. The anesthesiologist leaves but tells you that he is glad he is leaving, as he is very sleepy.

You sit down and start chartering. However, you notice that there is a smell of isoflurane in and around your anesthesia machine. You disconnect the carbon dioxide anesthetic agent sampling tube from the patient's breathing system. The tube is used to "sniff" for any possible leak of isoflurane. You "sniff" the anesthetic circuit tubing from the patient's endotracheal tube (ETT) to the machine and around the vaporizer but cannot find any evidence of a leak [1]. Accidentally you drop the sampling tube on the floor and 0.25 % isoflurane concentration is recorded on your Datex capnograph machine. You are at a loss to understand where the leak comes from.

Question

What can the problem be?

J.G. Brock-Utne, *Near Misses in Pediatric Anesthesia*,
DOI 10.1007/978-1-4614-7040-3_71, © Springer Science+Business Media New York 2013

Solution

You look at the waste gas scavenging system and discover that the waste anesthetic gas (WAG) outlet tubing is disconnected and lying on the floor. It is not attached to the outlet pipe that takes the WAG to the roof.

Discussion

When I started training in Oslo, Norway, in 1970 we did not have any scavenging systems. We did not have absorber systems in most operating rooms, so using Mapleson A systems and no scavenging led to an excessive amount of halothane in the operating room (OR) air. My wife could always tell if I had been in the OR, since she could smell the halothane coming from my skin after a long day in the OR.

Advances in waste gas scavenging systems, anesthesia delivery systems, decreased fresh gas flow, and awareness of OR environmental factors have decreased the risk of exposure to potentially harmful substances, such as nitrous oxide and anesthetic vapors.

In a previous study [2], we detected concentrations of sevoflurane within 67 s, 6 in. (15 cm) from the disconnected WAG outlet tubing.

In the Dräger Apollo workstation, there is another reason why you can get contamination of the OR environment. The waste gases go into a 3-gallon size container, but the gases are only emptied into the WAG outlet in the wall if suction is applied to the container. When there is no suction, the waste gases will passively leak out of the canister through holes on top of the canister and enter the room. So besides checking that the WAG outlet tubing is connected, you must also check that the suction for the WAG container is on. It is interesting that there are no locking mechanisms on the WAG tube, nor is there an alarm to indicate that the suction is not on.

The "sniff technique" has also been recommended as an adjuvant to the cuff-leak test [3].

Recommendation

1. A locking mechanism and a disconnect alarm should be installed on the WAG tubing.
2. A suction alarm should be installed, alarming when the suction in the WAG container is not on. These two recommendations (1 and 2) would be of considerable importance to reduce the risks of exposure to volatile anesthetic and nitrous oxide, thereby making the anesthetic machine in compliance with National Institute for Occupational Safety and Health (NIOSH) standards.
3. If you are feeling unusually tired during an anesthetic, make sure that you are not also being anesthetized by WAG.

References

1. Bolton P, Brock-Utne JG, Zumaran AA, Cummings J, Armstrong D. A simple method to identify an external vaporizer leak (the "sniff" method). Anesth Analg. 2005;101:606–7.
2. Reid CS, Brun C, Brock-Utne JG. No laughing matter: inadvertent exposure to waste anesthetic gas due to machine failure. Is there a solution? American Society of Anesthesiologist Annual meeting 15–19 Oct 2011, Chicago.
3. Eng MR, Wu TT, Brock-Utne JG. An adjuvant of the cuff leak test. Anaesthesia. 2009;64:452.

Chapter 72
Case 72: Check Your Facts

You are a senior attending anesthesiologist in a large private hospital. It is 6:40 a.m. One of your junior colleagues tells you about an 18-year-old patient who is to undergo laparoscopic laparotomy for an acute appendix. He is concerned as the patient has aortic stenosis with a valve area of < 0.7 mm. You tell him what to watch out for and which monitors to use. Your colleague is grateful for your comments and is seen taking the patient back to the operating room (OR) # 9 at 7:20 a.m.

Since your first case that morning is canceled, you are sitting in the OR doctors' lounge. At about 7:50 a.m., a code is heard from OR #9. You enter the darkened room where the surgery has begun. Your colleague is under the drapes by the side of the aortic stenosis patient's head. He is inserting a central line. You note a normal arterial waveform but the arterial systolic blood pressure is 50 mmHg. The arterial transducer is at the level of the heart. The patient is supine with both arms secured alongside the patient's body. The table is level. The noninvasive BP is cycling. The heart rate is 120 beats per minute (bpm) sinus rhythm and the oxygen saturation is 96 %. The left superficial temporal artery has a good pulse.

You ask, "How can I help?"

You are told that "The BP has suddenly dropped and now is 50 mmHg systolic; 1,000 mcg of epinephrine has been given with no effect on the BP."

You are asked by your colleague to kindly give the patient more intravenous (IV) epinephrine, which is lying on the back table.

Question

You see the epinephrine syringe and take it to the patient's IV injection port, but should you give it? Or what will you do?

J.G. Brock-Utne, *Near Misses in Pediatric Anesthesia*,
DOI 10.1007/978-1-4614-7040-3_72, © Springer Science+Business Media New York 2013

Solution

You squeeze the flush on the transducer—Transpac IV monitoring kit 84″ dispos-able transducer with a 3-ml squeeze flush (Abbott Critical Care system, Abbott Laboratory, North Chicago, IL)—with no effect on the waveform. You discover that the pressure bag attached to the transducer system has a very low pressure. You pump up the pressure bag, flush the system, and discover to your dismay that the arterial BP is 235/115 mmHg. At that moment, the noninvasive BP gives you a similar reading. You thank your lucky stars that you did not give any more epinephrine.

Discussion

Always check your facts. In this case, our colleague decided that the reason for the sudden low BP was related to his severe aortic stenosis. Hence, he opened the IVs, gave epinephrine, and called a code. Never jump to conclusions. It was indeed lucky that more epinephrine was not given. A dangerously high increase in BP could have led to a potentially bad outcome for the patient. In this case, the operation was con-cluded uneventfully and the patient woke up fully intact. Another cause of a func-tioning arterial line becoming a straight line or "dampened" (the magnitude of the difference between the input pressure and the transfused pressure) has been reported [1]. In that case, a nurse was securing wires from an operating room microscope alongside an anesthetized patient. Unfortunately, the clamp she used inadvertently clamped shut the radial artery line.

Recommendation

Always check the patient's pulses and vital signs before giving any drugs. In this case, it was obviously important to check the arterial transducer system.

Do not just do as you are told or asked to do. In this case, another pair of eyes prevented the patient from getting an excessive and potentially dangerous BP rise.

Reference

1. Truelsen KS, Brock-Utne JG. Damping of an arterial line: an unlikely cause. Anesth Analg. 1998;87:979–80.

Chapter 73
Case 73: A Strange Capnogram

You are an attending anesthesiologist in a large university hospital covering two operating rooms. In both rooms, you are working with very keen and enthusiastic residents. In one room is a 10-year-old female (American Society of Anesthesiologists physical status I [ASA 1] and 28 kg) who is given a routine general anesthetic (propofol and fentanyl) for an open reduction and internal fixation (ORIF) of the right ankle. She last ate 6 h ago. A ProSeal laryngeal airway (PLMA) (LMA Company Ltd. Mahe, Seychelles) (size 2.5) is placed without any problems. Vecuronium (4 mg) is given and mechanical ventilation is started. Two liters of FGF (fresh gas flow) (oxygen 50 %, nitrous oxide 50 % and isoflurane 0.6 %) is delivered and the peak pressure is 15 cm H_2O. Bilateral air entry, chest movement, and a normal capnograph waveform are seen (Fig. 73.1). The vital signs are stable.

A gastric suction catheter is passed successfully via the PLMA drainage tube, as seen by aspiration of gastric contents. At this point, you are called to your other room but return 15 min later to find the patient's vital signs are all in order. Your resident has placed a nasopharyngeal temperature probe (NTP) (DeRoyal, Powell, TN 37849) in the pharynx via the left nostril. You tell the resident to go to lunch and sit down to do your chartering. Now you notice for the first time that the capnogram has changed to a different waveform (Fig. 73.2).

J.G. Brock-Utne, *Near Misses in Pediatric Anesthesia*,
DOI 10.1007/978-1-4614-7040-3_73, © Springer Science+Business Media New York 2013

Fig. 73.1 A normal
capnograph waveform

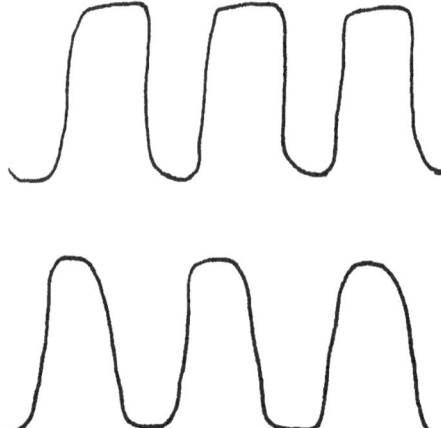

Fig. 73.2 An abnormal
capnograph waveform

Question

What is the cause of the change in the capnograph tracing and what will you do?

Solution

Remove the NTP and the waveform reverts to its previous size and shape. The NTP had produced a small leak.

Discussion

In a previous case report [1], after the NTP was introduced, the ventilator bellows collapsed. A leak could be heard coming from the mouth. When the NTP was withdrawn, the leak disappeared and the capnograph reverted to normal. It was postulated by the authors [1] that the absence of a dorsal cuff in the pediatric ProSeal could have led to the leak. The authors [1] speculate that if the intracuff pressure had been increased, the leak would have gone away. However, increases in intracuff pressures are not without concerns [2]. Personally, I never put anything in the nose unless I have to. I have seen too many epistaxis from placing tubes, etc., in the nose. One epistaxis was so serious that the child lost nearly half its blood volume before the ENT surgeon got control. Galante et al. [3] have recommended using the PLMA when a transesophageal Doppler probe is to be used in pediatric patients. The latter is inserted into the esophagus behind the PLMA. However to prevent oropharyngeal leak, the PLMA cuff had to be inflated to 60 cm H_2O. Uda [4] inserted a similar probe through the drainage port of the PLMA, but in pediatric PLMA the drainage port internal diameter will prove to be too small.

Recommendation

A temperature probe inserted either through the nose or mouth into the pharynx can cause an airway leak and change in the capnograph tracing when an LMA is used. If a leak is seen after a temperature probe is placed, then it should be removed and an alternate site for temperature monitoring should be used.

I always recommend using the drainage port on the ProSeal for your temperature probe.

References

1. Elakkumnan LB, Rewari V, Khanna P. An unusual cause for oropharyngeal leak during use of a 2.5 size ProSeal LMA. Pediatr Anesth. 2008;18:1229–30.
2. Brimacombe J, Keller C, Puhringer F. Pharyngeal mucosal pressure and perfusion: a fiberoptic evaluation of the posterior pharynx in anesthetized adult patients with a modified cuffed oropharyngeal airway. Anesthesiology. 1999;91:1661–5.
3. Galante D, Dambroiso M, Cinnella G. A new technique for the concurrent use of both ProSeal laryngeal mask airway and the transesophageal Doppler probe in pediatric patients. Pediatr Anesth. 2009;19:76–7.
4. Uda R. Versatility of the LMA-ProSeal for probe passage. Anesthesiology. 2002;96:1033.

Chapter 74
Case 74: Relying on Others

Today you are anesthetizing a patient who is morbidly obese—body mass index (BMI) 45—with acromegaly in the Magnetic resonance imaging (MRI) suite. The oxygen pipeline inside the MRI suite cannot reach outside the MRI and there is no piped oxygen in the preinduction room. Hence, the emergency oxygen tank, attached to the anesthesia machine (Aestiva, Datex Ohmeda) is used. In the preinduction room outside the MRI, the patient is ramped up and positioned for tracheal intubation [1, 2]. A rapid sequence induction is used with fentanyl, propofol, and succinylcholine and cricoid pressure. A grade 2 view is seen on laryngoscopy with a Mac 4 blade. After successful endotracheal intubation, bilateral air entry is heard and end-tidal carbon dioxide (CO_2) is seen. The endotracheal tube (ETT) is secured at 25 cm.

After the patient is anesthetized, he is rolled with the anesthesia machine into the MRI suite. The technician volunteers to supply the anesthetic machine with oxygen from the large "H" oxygen cylinder stationed in the MRI. You agree and see him attach the oxygen supply tubing from the anesthesia machine to the "H" oxygen cylinder.

With the patient anesthetized, ventilated appropriately, and with the vital signs stable you leave the room and the procedure begins. Five minutes later, sitting in the control room (outside the MRI suite), you notice that the end-tidal CO_2 and the tidal volume decreases dramatically over 45 s. All other vital signs are stable.

You tell the technician to stop the scan and rush into the MRI suite. You see that the patient is not being ventilated by the machine and switch to manual ventilation. You attempt unsuccessfully to manually ventilate the patient using the anesthesia machine. The reservoir bag remains empty, even though the adjustable pressure limiting (APL) value is closed and you are activating the emergency oxygen supply.

Question

What can the problem be and what will you do?

J.G. Brock-Utne, *Near Misses in Pediatric Anesthesia*,
DOI 10.1007/978-1-4614-7040-3_74, © Springer Science+Business Media New York 2013

Solution

The reason for the dilemma was that the Aestiva emergency oxygen cylinder was empty and the "H" oxygen cylinder was not turned on. Hence, no oxygen was flowing from the cylinder to the anesthesia machine.

Discussion

The MRI technician had attached the oxygen pipeline from the anesthetic machine to the "H" oxygen cylinder but he had not turned it on. When the anesthetic machine's only oxygen supply from the emergency tank became empty, the anesthesia machine ventilator (run by the oxygen) stopped functioning. This happened to me but luckily no changes to the vital signs were seen and the rest of the anesthetic was uneventful.

Recommendation

If you have to rely on others or ask others to do your job, then it is imperative that you check that things are done correctly. Not doing that can lead to a potential disaster.

References

1. Brodsky JB, Lemmens HJM, Brock-Utne JG, Vierra M, Saidman LJ. Morbid obesity and tracheal intubation. Anesth Analg. 2002;94:732–6.
2. Collins JS, Lemmens HJM, Brodsky JB, Brock-Utne JG, Levitan RM. Laryngoscopy and morbid obesity: a comparison of the "sniff" and "ramped" position. Obes Surg. 2004;14:1171–5.

Chapter 75
Case 75: Monitored Anesthesia Care. Watch Out

Today you are anesthetizing an 18-year-old girl (American Society of Anesthesiologists physical status I [ASA 1], 72 kg) for an orthopedic procedure. Her sister aged 28, who is accompanying her, has convinced the patient to have an epidural. The older sister has had two labor epidurals and claims, "They are the best thing since Swiss Cheese." You explain the options she has beside epidurals and outline the advantages, disadvantages, and risks of each one. The patient still wants an epidural. You explain to her that you will place the epidural in the operating room (OR) and give her sedation and keep an eye on her. You tell her this is called monitored anesthesia care (MAC).

You place an intravenous (IV) line and after 2 mg of midazolam you take the patient back to the OR where an epidural at L3-4 is placed without any problems. The epidural works very well, and a tourniquet is placed on her left calf. She states she does not want any more sedation and is seen happily lying there. You agree and give her no more IV sedation. Her vital signs are normal.

She occasionally asks, "What are they doing now?"

Oxygen is provided to the patient from the anesthesia machine fresh gas outlet (FGO) via a face mask. There is no separate oxygen outlet on this machine, hence the FGO is used.

After 10 min, your pal George from the bioengineering department in the hospital comes into your room. He is doing the routine check on all the vaporizers in the hospital. Since you are not using the vaporizers, he gets to work. You move out of his way and are now sitting on the patient's left side. The patient is closest to the anesthesia machine. George discovers that the sevoflurane vaporizer output is too low and replaces it with a new one. He leaves. Twenty minutes later, the patient begins to snore and her jaw needs to be supported. You diagnose the soporific effects of sensor de-afferentiation caused by the epidural. Still sitting on the left side of the patient, you place a finger between the rami of her mandible. Another 10 min go by and she seems to be even more asleep than before. You also seem to smell sevoflurane in the air and take that to mean that George spilt some sevoflurane when he replaced the vaporizer.

J.G. Brock-Utne, *Near Misses in Pediatric Anesthesia*,
DOI 10.1007/978-1-4614-7040-3_75, © Springer Science+Business Media New York 2013

Question

Should you be concerned that the patient is so sleepy? If so, what will you do?

Solution

You turn your attention to the anesthesia machine and note to your horror that George has inadvertently left the sevoflurane vaporizer on 4 %. You had not noticed that the patient was getting a high concentration of sevoflurane via the face mask. Remember that the oxygen was provided to the patient from the anesthesia machine fresh gas outlet (FGO) via the face mask. There was no separate oxygen outlet on this machine, hence the FGO is used.

The vaporizer was turned off and the patient over 3–4 min recovers consciousness and states, "This is so cool."

Discussion

This has happened to me. It is imperative to keep an eye on your anesthesia machine, even as in this case you are not "using it." This is especially true if others are working on it while you are providing anesthesia care. It is so easy to get lulled into a false sense of security if you provide just a MAC.

Recommendation

Vigilance is as important during MAC as it is during general anesthesia (GA).

Chapter 76
Case 76: An Intermittently Worrisome Capnography Trace

A routine general anesthetic is in progress. The child is 10 years old (American Society of Anesthesiologists physical status I [ASA1], 33 kg) undergoing an orthopedic procedure. He is being ventilated through an endotracheal tube (ETT) with N_2O 70 % in oxygen and sevoflurane using the circle system attached to an Apollo machine (Dräger Medical Inc., Telford, PA). The soda lime in the canister has just been replaced prior to the start of this anesthetic. The fresh gas flow (FGF) is 2 L/min.

Thirty minutes into the case, you see an intermittent capnograph tracing over a 3–4-min period (Fig. 76.1).

You confirm adequate ventilation as seen by observation and auscultation. The vital signs are normal and have not changed.

J.G. Brock-Utne, *Near Misses in Pediatric Anesthesia*,
DOI 10.1007/978-1-4614-7040-3_76, © Springer Science+Business Media New York 2013

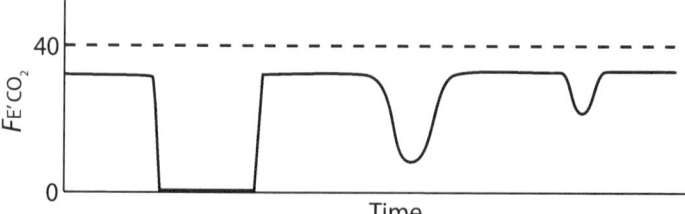

Fig. 76.1 Diagram of capnography trace showing development of rebreathing pattern. Modified with permission from Parry TM, Jewkes DA, Smith M. A sticking flutter valve. Anaesthesia. 1991;46(3):229

Question

What can the problem be?

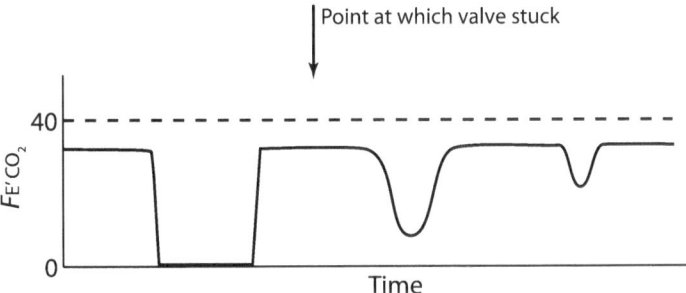

Fig. 76.2 Diagram of capnograph trace showing development of rebreathing pattern subsequent to sticking of flutter valve. Modified with permission from Parry TM, Jewkes DA, Smith M. A sticking flutter valve. Anaesthesia. 1991;46(3):229

Solution

A sticking flutter valve on the expiratory limb of the circle system is intermittently in the open position [1] (Fig. 76.2). This causes significant rebreathing resulting in the abnormal capnograph tracing (Fig. 76.1). Since it was intermittent and the duration short, a rise in end-tidal CO_2 was not seen.

Discussion

When a flutter valve in a circle system gets stuck, it can lead to retention of CO_2. In this case the valve closure was intermittent, preventing a rise in the end-tidal CO_2 concentration. Without the capnography, the faulty valve would have not been detected. This could have led to an increase in end-tidal CO_2 and arterial CO_2. The latter could have risen to dangerous levels.

Recommendation

Your routine check of the vital signs should always include a look at the waveform of the capnopraphy. Any change could signal the beginning of a potential clinical problem.

Reference

1. Parry TM, Jewkes DA, Smith M. A sticking flutter valve. Anaesthesia. 1991;46(3):229.

Chapter 77
Case 77: Cardiac Arrest at the Conclusion of Neurosurgery

Today you are anesthetizing an 8-month-old child (6 kg) who is otherwise healthy, for closure of craniosynostosis. Routine inhalational induction is done after all monitors are placed on the child. While the child is asleep, an intravenous (IV) line is established and a rocuronium 5 mg is given. The trachea is intubated successfully. Anesthesia is maintained with isoflurane 0.6–1.1 % in 50 % N$_2$O in oxygen. Fentanyl 4 mcg and morphine 0.1 mg/kg is given. There is no problem until closure of the skin. At that time, reversal was given and the child started to breath spontaneously. The arterial blood gas, serum electrolytes, and coagulation profiles, taken an hour ago, are normal. Suddenly there is a decrease of the HR to 60 beats per minute (bpm) from 115 bpm and an increase of the BP to 140/80 from 90/60.

Question

What is going on and what will you do?

J.G. Brock-Utne, *Near Misses in Pediatric Anesthesia*, 241
DOI 10.1007/978-1-4614-7040-3_77, © Springer Science+Business Media New York 2013

Solution

Inform the surgeon that there is a risk of increased intracranial pressure (ICP) as seen by the presence of a Cushing reflex. The surgeon should consider reopening the scalp sutures.

In this case, blood had collected under the flap and caused an increase in ICP. The flap was removed. The child's vital signs stabilized with ventilation with 100 % oxygen and IV atropine. The child made an uneventful recovery.

Discussion

The Cushing reflex has been described as bradycardia, hypertension, and apnea following sudden increase in ICP [1, 2]. Heymans [3] refined the findings above, showing a short-lived initial tachycardia and hypertension prior to the onset of the reflex. The Cushing reflex has been described during closure of a craniosynostosis repair [3]. In these cases, a sudden life-threatening intracranial hypertension can occur. Sometimes at the end of a neurosurgical case, with the patient breathing spontaneously, the Cushing reflex can occur for another reason. In patients with moderately raised intracranial pressure, the ICP may rise dangerously high, at the end of the anesthetic, due to inadequate ventilation. Even a relatively small increase in CO_2 will cause the ICP to rise. If the vital signs in the above case had changed to severe bradycardia and hypotension, then one must look at the subcutaneous wound drain and its container. The surgeons have a habit of hiding it. Several times, I have found the container to be full of blood when the child suddenly has become bradycardic and hypotensive. Again, the surgeon must be encouraged to open the wound and stop the venous bleeding.

Recommendation

Cushing reflex, if not diagnosed and potentially treated, can lead to a bad outcome in the immediate postoperative period.

References

1. Cushing H. Concerning a definite regulatory mechanism of the vasomotor center which controls blood pressure during cerebral compression. John Hopkins Hosp Bull. 1901;12:290–2.
2. Cushing H. The blood pressure reaction of acute cerebral compression, illustrated by cases of intracranial hemorrhage. Am J Med Sci. 1903;125:1017–44.
3. Erol DD. A risk of during an elective repair of craniosynostosis: the Cushing reflex. Pediatr Anesth. 2006;17:496–502.

Chapter 78
Case 78: Watch Out

It is early on a Saturday morning. The surgeon has booked an emergency tracheostomy in the operating room (OR). The patient is a 12-year-old girl. She has been in the intensive care unit (ICU) for the last week following a head injury. There are no associated injuries. On arrival in the OR she is sedated, intubated, and ventilated. Her vital signs are stable. You attach her to your OR monitors and anesthesia machine ventilator. The surgeon, who is in a hurry, is seen using diathermy for the dissection of the trachea. As he is about to cut (using diathermy) into the trachea, he tells you to pull the endotracheal tube (ETT) back. You instruct your resident to let some air out of the ETT cuff and to pull the ETT back but not out of the trachea.

Question

Is there anything wrong with this picture?

Solution

Never let a surgeon open the trachea with diathermy. That should only be done with a scalpel. Several cases have been reported [1–3] of the ETT cuff being ignited during tracheostomy by electrocautery.

Discussion

In the above case, a loud explosion was heard as the surgeon made an incision with diathermy into the trachea. The ETT was immediately removed and a tracheostomy tube was inserted without any problems. Examination of the cuff on the ETT showed that the cuff had exploded [1]. Sosis and Braverman [4] recommend the use of 20–30 % oxygen in air or helium during general anesthesia for tracheostomy. Nitrous oxide should not be used as it supports combustion. Others have suggested that the air in the cuff be replaced with saline to reduce the incidence of tracheal tube fires [5]. Never take the ETT out of the trachea until the surgeon has secured the airway with a tracheostomy tube (TT). The ETT should not be removed from the trachea until the TT is seen to be working. This is done in case the surgeon loses the airway. Should the airway not be secured by the surgeon, then you can rapidly push your ETT down into the trachea and inflate the cuff.

Recommendation

Never let a surgeon use diathermy when making the tracheal incision during tracheostomy. Fires and explosions can be a disaster for the patient.

References

1. Michels AMJ, Stott S. Explosion of tracheal tube during tracheostomy. Anaesthesia. 1994;49:1104.
2. Le Chair J, Gartner S, Halma G. Endotracheal tube cuff ignited by electrocautery during tracheostomy. Am Assoc Nurse Anesth. 1990;58:259–61.
3. Bailey MK, Bromley HR, Allison JG. Electrocautery induced airway fire during tracheostomy. Anesth Analg. 1990;71:702–4.
4. Sosis MB, Braverman B. Prevention of cautery-induced airway fires with special endotracheal tubes. Anesth Analg. 1993;77:846–7.
5. Sosis MB, Dillon FX. Saline-filled cuffs help prevent laser induced polyvinylchloride endotracheal tube fires. Anesth Analg. 1991;72:187–9.

Chapter 79
Case 79: A Complication of Central Venous Cannulation?

Today you are scheduled to anesthetize a 5.5-year-old boy (20 kg) for bone marrow aspiration, lumbar puncture, and insertion of a subclavian vein cannula. He was diagnosed with acute lymphatic leukemia but now he was having a relapse. He is otherwise healthy except for a platelet count of 20,000. Prior to the anesthetic, he is transfused with platelets and his count improves to 90,000.

A routine inhalation anesthetic is given and maintained with 50 % nitrous oxide in oxygen and sevoflurane. The patient is kept breathing spontaneously with a face mask. The lumbar puncture and the bone marrow aspiration, with the patient in the lateral and supine positions, respectively, are done without any incidence.

In preparation for the subclavian vein cannulation via the infraclavicular route, the patient is placed in Trendelenburg (25°). The cannulation proves difficult. During the third attempt, the patient's heart rate suddenly increases from 110 to a sinus tachycardia of 165 beats per minute (bpm) and his breathing became labored and noisy. The oxygen saturation falls to 96 %. The subclavian attempt is stopped. The mask is removed and much to your horror you see fresh pink blood freely flowing from his nose and mouth.

Leaving the child in Trendelenburg, you turn him onto his left lateral position and insert a laryngoscope. To your surprise, no blood is coming from the laryngeal opening. But there is a steady flow of blood seen in the posterior nasal space. With 100 % oxygen from the face mask and the patient breathing spontaneously, his vital signs improve to oxygen saturation of 98 % and the heart rate decreases to 150 bpm.

Question

What can the problem be and what will you do?

J.G. Brock-Utne, *Near Misses in Pediatric Anesthesia*,
DOI 10.1007/978-1-4614-7040-3_79, © Springer Science+Business Media New York 2013

Solution

A spontaneous nose bleed. This occurred because of the high venous pressure generated by the Trendelenburg together with the sudden onset of sinus tachycardia and the qualitative deficiency in platelet function and/or capillary fragility.

Discussion

This complication has been previously described [1]. The hemorrhage in the above case gradually stopped over a 5-min period with the patient in Trendelenburg. The patient recovered fully without incidence. At a later date he underwent the subclavian cannulation after having been given more platelets, preoperative packing of the nose, and a less steep Trendelenburg. Initially the authors [1] thought that they had hit the tracheobronchial tree with their subclavian needle. This has, as far as I can ascertain, never been reported.

Recommendation

Epistaxis may occur, when patients, who are at risk from spontaneous bleeding, are placed in the Trendelenburg position.

Reference

1. Thomas DG, Bray BM. Complication of central venous cannulation. Anaesthesia. 1986;41:769.

Chapter 80
Case 80: An Example of Murphy's Law

Today you are in the intensive care unit (ICU) as the attending anesthesiologist. It is late at night. A 17-year-old female has been ventilated for several days, following a motor vehicle accident (MVA). You notice that the patient is now requiring high inflation pressures to maintain her oxygenation. Copious amount of purulent sputum are sucked out of her endotracheal tube (ETT) with minimal improvement in the peak airway pressures.

You place a bronchoscopic swivel adaptor (PriMedico, Largo, FL) to the proximal (patient) end of the ETT. The swivel is useful, as it allows ventilation during the bronchoscopy [1]. Through the swivel you pass a well-lubricated flexible fiber-optic bronchoscope down the patient's ETT. This is done to examine the tracheobronchial tree. The ETT is seen to be full of secretions. The carina and right-side bronchi are visualized and, with the exception of moderate amount of purulent sputum, no other abnormality is seen. However when you attempt to withdraw the bronchoscope to examine the left side, you are unsuccessful because you feel significant resistance. Interestingly you discover that you can advance the scope, but any attempt to remove it is futile.

You decide to let the patient's ETT cuff down and remove both the ETT and the scope at the same time. With the ETT removed, you quickly reinsert a new ETT into her trachea and commence ventilation.

Questions

1. What can the cause be for this dilemma?
2. What would you do if the patient had a previously difficult intubation?

Solution

This happened to a great friend of mine, Rob MacGillivray [2]. He called his case report: "Eye to eye with Murphy's Law" [2, 3]. Most appropriate. The problem was that the scope, instead of leaving the ETT at its distal end, left the ETT through the Murphy's eye. This was probably caused by the large amount of purulent secretions in the distal end of the ETT diverting the thin fiber-optic scope out of the Murphy's eye. Having gone through the "eye" the scope got stuck and although the scope could advance, it could not be removed. By removing the ETT and the scope together at the same time, neither the patient nor the instrument was harmed.

Discussion

In this case, the management was correct. However, had this been a difficult intubation, a second fiber-optic bronchoscope (loaded with an ETT) would have had to be placed in the trachea. In these cases, an ENT surgeon should be at the ready for a potential emergency tracheostomy.

Murphy's eye was first described in 1941[4], but ETTs with Murphy's eyes did not become available until much later. The hole in the bevel of the ETT (Murphy's eye) was invented to allow ventilation of gas to pass out of the ETT should the main outlet of the ETT be occluded. The occlusion of the main outlet could be caused by the wall of the trachea or by any other obstruction. In old anesthesia textbooks (1940–1970), pictures of patients, with an ETT placed, show the tube always secured on the left side of the mouth. This was done to prevent the distal outlet of the ETT from coming up against the wall of the trachea and obstructing the airflow.

Recommendation

This is an uncommon complication, but should it prove impossible to remove the scope, then both the ETT and the scope must be taken out together. However, before you take out the ETT, you must ascertain that you can secure the airway after the ETT has been removed.

References

1. Torralva PR, Macario A, Brock-Utne JG. Another use of the bronchoscopic swivel adaptor. Anesth Analg. 1999;88:1187–8.
2. MacGillivray RG, Odell JA. Eye to eye with Murphy's law. Anaesthesia. 1986;41:334.
3. Bloch A. Murphy's law – "If anything can go wrong, it will". In: Murphy's law – and other reasons why things go wrong. Los Angeles: Price, Stern & Sloan; 1977.
4. Murphy FJ. Two improved intratracheal catheters. Anesth Analg. 1941;20:102–5.

Chapter 81
Case 81: A Tragic Case

Today you find yourself in the labor delivery suite (LD). A previously fit and healthy 19-year-old female (74 kg, gravida 1, para 0) is admitted to the LD. She is 34 weeks pregnant and is complaining of an increasingly severe headache and left-sided facial weakness. At 28 weeks, she had been admitted to the emergency room (ER) after a witnessed grand mal epileptic convulsion. Investigations showed an extensive right frontoparietal lesion. The diagnosis is suggestive of a glioma. It was decided that she should be started on Phenytoin and be allowed to continue her pregnancy.

Today her vital signs are normal but she is very drowsy. Her retina shows papilledema. The obstetrician suggests an elective Cesarean section and the patient concurs. Before anyone can discuss with her the anesthetic technique, the patient says she really would like to have a vaginal delivery under epidural.

Questions

What do you think? Good idea or bad idea?

J.G. Brock-Utne, *Near Misses in Pediatric Anesthesia*,
DOI 10.1007/978-1-4614-7040-3_81, © Springer Science+Business Media New York 2013

Solution

A general anesthetic, not a regional block, is advisable.

Discussion

In a previous case [1], a 23-year-old primigravida with an inoperable frontal glioma was given a general anesthetic. The mother and child were discharged home, but the mother died 4 weeks later. There are cases in the literature [2, 3] where either caudal or epidural were used successfully in managing such cases. The main reason for using regional anesthesia is that, in experienced hands, the incidence of dural puncture is very low [4, 5]. These authors quote a rate between 2 % and 3 % in obstetrical patients without a raised intracranial pressure. The other reason that a regional block is not a good idea is that lumbar epidural injection of local anesthetic, or saline, increases intracranial pressure (ICP). The ICP increase is greater, if intracranial pressure is already high [6]. These authors [6] recommend that epidural anesthesia should be used with extreme caution in patients with reduced intracranial compliance and should not be used at all in patients with intracranial hypertension or a space-occupying lesion.

Recommendation

Regional anesthesia would seem to be less appropriate than general anesthesia in these cases.

References

1. Chater SN, Greig AJ, Sugden JC. Epidural anesthesia in the presence of a cerebral tumour. Anaesthesia. 1987;42:443.
2. Keps ER, Andrews C, Radnay PA, Schapira M, Stark DCC. Conduct of anesthesia for delivery with grossly raised cerebro-spinal fluid pressure. N Y State J Med. 1972;72:1155–6.
3. Goroszeniuk T, Howard RS, Wright JT. The management of labour using continuous lumbar epidural analgesia in a patient with a malignant cerebral tumour. Anaesthesia. 1986;41:1128–9.
4. Hodgkinson R. Total spinal block after epidural injection into an interspace adjacent to an inadvertent dural perforation. Anesthesiology. 1981;55:593–5.
5. Moir DD, Thorburn J. Obstetric anaesthesia and analgesia. 3rd ed. London: Baillière Tindall; 1986. 238.
6. Hilt H, Gramm HJ, Link J. Changes in intracranial pressure associated with extradural anaesthesia. BJA. 1986;58:676–80.

Chapter 82
Case 82: Hemoptysis from a 2-Month Tracheostomy

You are called to the emergency room (ER). A 19-year-old male (1.6 m and 63 kg) is complaining that he had over half a cup of acute bright red hemoptysis from his tracheostomy site in the last hour. The patient has a 3-day history of blood-tinged sputum from the tracheostomy site. He is in remission from a non-Hodgkin's lymphoma for which he has received chemotherapy and radiation with good effect. He had required a tracheostomy because of severe swelling of face and neck with acute airway obstruction. A computed tomography angiography (CTA) of the neck and chest has been done while in the ER, and is negative for any active bleeding.

The ENT surgeon is at the bedside and you are asked to provide sedation for a fiber-optic bronchoscopy. This is to be done in the ER. You examine the patient and concur with giving the patient midazolam. He receives up to 3 mg with good effect. The vital signs remain stable. The surgeon examines the trachea with a flexible fiber-optic scope through the patient 6.0 mm Moore tracheostomy tube. The tracheostomy tube is seen sitting on and irritating the carina. There is no sign of active bleeding. The surgeon is unable to examine the rest of the airway, due to bloody secretions and because the patient is distressed and coughing a lot. The fiber-optic scope is removed and the patient settles down. A little later, the ENT physician removes the patient's tracheostomy tube. The distal part of the tube is cut down by 1.5 cm. The tube is then repositioned in the trachea. The patient is sent home but booked the next morning for a flexible bronchoscopy under general anesthesia in the operating room.

You are the anesthesiologist who is going to anesthetize him the next day. The surgeon informs you that he will remove the tracheostomy tube after the patient has been anesthetized. You are to replace the tracheostomy tube with an endotracheal tube (ETT) through the tracheostomy for oxygenation and anesthesia. The surgeon then plans to do a fiber-optic bronchoscopy through the ETT.

J.G. Brock-Utne, *Near Misses in Pediatric Anesthesia*,
DOI 10.1007/978-1-4614-7040-3_82, © Springer Science+Business Media New York 2013

Questions

Does this sound like a plan? Or what will you suggest? Would you do a monitored anesthesia care (MAC) or a general anesthesia (GA)?

Solution

This is not a good idea. The placement of the ETT will hinder the surgeon's ability to locate the source of bleeding, should the bleeding come from the trachea above the end of the ETT tube.

The bronchoscopy is done under sedation with the patient breathing spontaneously with the tracheostomy tube. Over a period of 40 min, the patient is given midazolam 2 mg and glycopyrrolate 0.4 mg. He is maintained on ketamine boluses during the 40-min procedure, receiving a total of 155 mg intravenous ketamine.

Discussion

Upon entry into the trachea through the tracheostomy tube, and with the patient breathing spontaneously, the ENT surgeon finds a significant amount of clot in the distal trachea that obstructed his view. In order to remove these, saline irrigation and suction is required. Inspection of the airways bilaterally past the bronchi revealed further bloody clots. This is also sucked out. At the end of the procedure, the tracheostomy tube is removed and the trachea inspected. The mucosa of the posterior wall of the trachea, opposite the tracheostomy site, is very friable, with some sign of arterial bleeding. Diathermy is used with good effect. However, ice-cold saline irrigation is required twice, as the first attempt at reinserting the tracheostomy tube causes recurrent oozing from the posterior wall of the trachea. After 5 min of observation in the operating room, the bleeding stops and the case is concluded. The patient is transported to the recovery room in a stable condition.

Recommendation

In these cases, it is imperative that the whole of the trachea is inspected for possible bleeding sites.

Chapter 83
Case 83: A Potentially Serious Incident

Today you are in the endoscopy suite. On entering the procedure room, you note that the anesthesia machine is an older version of the one you use in the rest of the hospital. You check the anesthesia machine and find everything is in order. There is piped oxygen into the procedure room and the emergency oxygen and nitrous oxide cylinders on the back of the machine are full. A large see-through plastic bag with an Ambu bag is hanging on the side of the anesthesia machine beside the absorber. You now recall that at a departmental morbidity and mortality (M&M) meeting there had been an incident of a sudden anesthesia machine failure in the endoscopy suite. You check the Ambu bag and find it in order. You ask that a separate full cylinder of oxygen be brought into the procedure room. This is to be used with the Ambu bag to provide a higher inspired oxygen concentration, in case the anesthesia machine stops functioning.

The child is a 2-year-old who is coming for upper and lower endoscopy for undiagnosed anemia. She is otherwise healthy. A routine general anesthetic is performed with an endotracheal tube. After about 10 min, you notice that the fresh gas flow has to be increased from 2 to 4 L (nitrous oxide 50 % in oxygen). A check for leaks or malfunction reveals nothing abnormal. The procedure is concluded after 45 min, but you are dismayed to note that it has been necessary to increase the fresh gas flow to 10 L a minute. There seems to be a leak, but you cannot find it. Throughout the anesthetic, the patient's vital signs were stable. At the end of the procedure, the patient is taken to the recovery room where she makes an uneventful recovery. She is discharged after 90 min.

Question

What can be the cause of the large leak?

J.G. Brock-Utne, *Near Misses in Pediatric Anesthesia*,
DOI 10.1007/978-1-4614-7040-3_83, © Springer Science+Business Media New York 2013

Solution

At the end of the procedure, the machine was checked and you discover that the plastic bag covering the Ambu bag had been sucked into the side of the active scavenging unit. The negative pressure that was generated emptied the gas in the patient's circuit.

Discussion

The hospital "active" scavenging unit operates continuously 24/7 at a nominally slow rate of 35–75 L/min from each operating room [1]. These units can be seen on the side of the anesthetic machines. As a safety feature, they have openings to the operating room. Negative pressure results if these openings are occluded. If that happens, the fresh gas that is intended for the patient will be sucked out and not delivered to the patient.

This case reminds one of the need for caution when using active scavenging systems. Hence, any plastic bags and the like must not be placed near these systems. Many hospitals do not employ active scavenging, but rather use a passive system. In those cases, a scavenging tube goes from the back of the machine to a wall socket.

Recommendation

Active scavenging systems are very useful, but if their openings to the room are obstructed, negative pressure will be created and the patient's fresh gas flow will decrease over time. If the suction is very strong, the gas flow to the patient can decrease rapidly, with potentially disastrous results.

Reference

1. Barwise JA, Lancaster LJ, Michaels D, Pope JE, Berry JM. An initial evaluation of a novel anesthetic scavenging interface. Anesth Analg. 2011;113:1064–7.

Chapter 84
Case 84: Rusty Material in an Oxygen Flowmeter

You are visiting a very good friend who is also an anesthesiologist. He lives in a part of the world where there is a yearly heavy rainfall. Your friend is on call and of course he gets called in. You accompany him to do a case late in the afternoon.

The case is a 9-month-old girl who is admitted to the emergency room (ER) with stridor and shortness of breath. She has a history of recurrent chest infections. The chest X-ray shows her trachea to be markedly displaced anteriorly and narrowed. Ultrasound showed a fluid-filled cyst in the mediastinum. Your friend is asked to provide general anesthesia for a scan. The scan is situated in the cellars of the hospital. Your colleague rightly wants to control the patient's airway prior to the transport to the scan. She is anesthetized and her trachea intubated in the ER. Her lungs are ventilated via a Mapleson F system (Jackson-Rees' modification of the Ayre's T-piece) attached to an oxygen cylinder. You note that the ER oxygen cylinder has a flowmeter on it and it is set at 8 l/min. She is transported to the scanner, paralyzed and sedated.

With a nurse you run to the scanner where you volunteer to check the anesthesia machine. Having completed your task, your friend and patient arrive in the scanner. Your pal suddenly says, "Look at this." To your amazement, you see some rust-colored fluid/material suddenly filling the flowmeter on the oxygen cylinder that is being used to ventilate the patient. The fluid/material pushes the bobbin upward and enters the fresh gas tubing to the Mapleson F system. Your friend quickly disconnects the Jackson-Rees from the patient and you help to roll the patient into the scanner. Here the patient is attached to the breathing circuit of the scanner's anesthesia machine. Luckily no rusty fluid was seen entering the patient's endotracheal tube. The scan was done uneventfully. A week later, a large bronchogenic cyst was removed.

Question

But what was the material in the flowmeter and tubing and how did it get there?

Solution

The material was rusty water.

Discussion

In a previous case report [1], the cylinder was sent to the manufacturer who dismantled it. They found the cylinder dry with no evidence of water having entered it. However, a film of rust had formed around the threads of the valve. The conclusion drawn was that the cylinder must have been left outside without a protective cap. They also stated that water was not removed from the valve outlet when the regulator was connected. The manufacturer concluded that if cylinders are to be stored in the open, then a cap must be placed and the cylinder stored on its side to minimize water getting to the valve.

I have seen this in a mission hospital in Africa. In a rudimentary anesthetic machine that ran on oxygen cylinders, the oxygen flowmeter got flooded with rusty water. An Ambu bag saved the day.

Recommendation

If oxygen cylinders must be stored outside, then a protective cap must be utilized. The cylinders should be stored on their side. It is also imperative to wipe down the threads of the valve should they be seen or felt to be moist.

Reference

1. Schiller DJ. Rusty water in an oxygen flow meter. Anaesthesia. 1986;41:1061.

Chapter 85
Case 85: A Surprising Solution to an Airway Emergency

A 19-year-old female (170 cm and 120 kg; body mass index [BMI] 41.5; American Society of Anesthesiologists physical status III [ASA 3]) is scheduled for a biliary stent removal in the endoscopy suite. Her past history consisted of hypertension, hyperlipidemia, anemia, end-stage renal disease on hemodialysis, and diabetes mellitus type 2. On exam she is noted to have a neck circumference of 60.5 cm.

She had undergone two procedures: an endoscopic retrograde cholangiopancreatography (ERCP) and a cholecystectomy recently. Both times she had been intubated successfully, albeit with difficulty, using an awake fiber-optic technique.

You decide to do the procedure under ketamine sedation. This is because you are told it will take less than 3 min and the senior gastroenterologist (whom you trust) is going to do the procedure.

The patient is placed in the left lateral position and the pharynx and the upper airway is sprayed with Cetacaine 200 mg. Thereafter, you give midazolam 1 mg, glycopyrrolate 0.4 mg, and ketamine 70 mg. The stent is successfully identified, but as it is removed the patient is suddenly desaturated with an upper airway obstructive pattern. You diagnose laryngospasm and commence mask ventilation. As expected, she is an extremely difficult mask airway and the oxygen saturation keeps falling to 84 % and beyond. The other vital signs have not changed significantly.

Question

Knowing that you will have great difficulty in quickly placing an endotracheal tube with a fiber-optic scope and even an LMA should an airway problem occur, what was your plan B?

Solution

We had a case like this [1]. Prior to the start of the procedure, we asked the endoscopist to prepare a smaller endoscope loaded with an endotracheal tube. Within 30 s after the diagnosis of laryngospam, the gastroenterologist had secured the airway using his endoscope. The patient was taken to the intensive care unit (ICU) to be monitored since her saturation had fallen to the mid 60s for a short period. Later that evening, she was extubated and transferred to the step-down unit. She made an uneventful recovery.

Recommendation

Remember if you are in trouble or think you may be in trouble with a patient's airway in the endo-suite, the endoscopist may be your friend in quickly finding the trachea.

Reference

1. Wang R. Brock-Utne JG. A surprising solution to an airway problem in the endoscopic suite. Western Anesthesia Residents conference, Albuquerque, New Mexico, 10 May 2013.

Chapter 86
Case 86: An Airway Leak in the ICU

A 16-year-old girl (85 kg, 5′ 2″) is on full ventilator support in the intensive care unit (ICU). She was involved in a motor vehicle accident (MVA) and has sustained multiple rib fractures with lung contusion, which necessitated endotracheal intubation. The ICU nurse tells you that the intubation proved difficult, but with a two-handed technique they were able to adequately oxygenate the patient. After several attempts, a bougie was blindly inserted into the trachea and the airway secured. It is now 1 h later and you are called because the nurse informs you that there is air coming out of the mouth on inspiration. The nurse tells you that the respiratory therapist had just increased the tidal volume. Vital signs are within normal limits, oxygen saturation 95 %, heart rate 105, and BP 130/80. You can hear air escaping from the patient's mouth. A #7 endotracheal tube (ETT) is taped at 22 cm and a nasogastric tube has been inserted. The latter is attached to continuous suction. The cuff on the pilot tubing feels full but you put in another 3–5 ml of air. The cuff now feels very tight. But there is no improvement in the air leak. The patient is covered with a blanket, which you remove to examine the chest. There is equal bilateral air entry and the chest is clear to auscultation. There is no evidence of surgical emphysema or pneumothorax. The peak pressure generated by the ventilator is 32 cm H_2O. An ETT suction catheter goes through the whole length of the ETT. There are no secretions in the trachea.

Since you do not know what else to do, you are about to exchange the existing ETT with a new ETT using a gum-elastic bougie [1].

Question

However, you suddenly realized that there is something you have not checked. What is that and what can the problem be?

J.G. Brock-Utne, *Near Misses in Pediatric Anesthesia*,
DOI 10.1007/978-1-4614-7040-3_86, © Springer Science+Business Media New York 2013

Solution

The nasogastric tube is found to be in the back of the mouth and not in the stomach. You examine the epigastrium and discover a dilated stomach from the mask ventilation prior to the insertion of the ETT into the trachea.

After the nasogastric tube is properly positioned and the stomach emptied for air, no further leak is heard.

Discussion

During a difficult intubation with mask ventilation an excessive amount of air can find its way into the stomach. This must be emptied with an oral or nasogastric tube; otherwise, you will get the problem described in this case. If not diagnosed, many would exchange the existing ETT for a new one using a tube changer. This would not improve the air leak but in exchange could cause the airway to be lost.

Recommendation

Both the chest and abdomen must be examined when confronted with a problem like this.

Reference

1. Robles B, Hester J, Brock-Utne JG. Remember the gum-elastic bougie at extubation. J Clin Anesth. 1993;5:329–31.

Chapter 87
Case 87: Pediatric Dental Anesthesia

Today you are doing a list of children for dental extractions. All the children have behavioral problems. The first child is a 10-year-old autistic boy. He is otherwise healthy. You suggest placing an intravenous (IV) line, but he becomes very agitated. You decide against an oral midazolam as a premedication as you have had several children with postoperative cognitive impairment [1]. This also includes this child. This impairment, although transient, led to the parents of these children being unhappy with your anesthetic management. They were worried that his impairment this time may be permanent.

Intramuscular ketamine is not an option; this is because the mother states that the last time her son had ketamine he was adversely affected by it for days. Since there is a drug shortage, you have no barbiturates to be given via rectum. You decide on an inhalational anesthetic induction and attempt a distraction technique. You tell him that he and you are going to go and blow up balloons. But he will have nothing to do with you. As is your usual practice in these cases, you ask the parent or parents to accompany you and the child to the procedure room [2, 3]. Your plan is to do an inhalational induction with sevoflurane. In the room, the child is being cuddled on the mother's lap. The room light is dimmed. Soft music is being played. You attempt to place an oxygen saturation probe, electrocardiogram (ECG) pads, and a blood pressure (BP) cuff on the child. But he will not have them anywhere near him.

Question

What trick do you know that may make the child have at least the oxygen saturation probe on his finger?

J.G. Brock-Utne, *Near Misses in Pediatric Anesthesia*,
DOI 10.1007/978-1-4614-7040-3_87, © Springer Science+Business Media New York 2013

Solution

You place the oxygen saturation probe on the mother's finger and the child sees the wavy line on the TV screen and the number. "Let's see if you can beat your mum's number." This usually works, as it becomes a game [4].

Discussion

Anesthetizing these very unfortunate children can be a great challenge. The anesthetic management of these cases depends on the age, size, and the demeanor of the child. The parent's behavior and understanding of what has to be done is also important. For the above trick to work, obviously the child has to understand and be able to read numbers. If the child cannot read numbers then he may be convinced to make bigger waves than his mum. It also helps to have two oxygen saturation monitors.

Flatt [5] suggests that the child try and breathe so deeply that he can beat 100. This he claims has worked very well. Bringing parents to the operating room has many advantages but also some disadvantages. One recently published case [6] talks of a mother who, after her child was anesthetized with a sevoflurane induction, picked the child up and tried to wake him up. In the process, all the monitoring equipment was disconnected. The child recovered and the procedure cancelled.

Recommendation

Being understanding and kind is a prerequisite in dealing with these children and their families, but being inventive is imperative.

References

1. Millar K, Asbury AJ, Bowman AW, Hosey MT, Martin K, Musiello T, Wellbury RR. A randomized placebo-controlled trial of the effects of midazolam premedication on children's' postoperative cognition. Anaesthesia. 2007;62:923–30.
2. Iacobucci T, Federico B, Pintus C, de Francisci G. Evaluation of satisfaction level by parents and children following pediatric anesthesia. Paediatr Anaesth. 2005;15:314–20.
3. Kain ZN, Maclaren J, Weinberg M, Huszti H, Anderson C, Mayes L. How many parents should we let into the operating room. Paediatr Anaesth. 2009;19:244–9.
4. Brock-Utne JG. A suggestion to help with anesthetizing mentally retarded children. Submitted for publication.
5. Flatt NW. Bribery in the anaesthesia room. Anaesthesia. 2007;62:1301.
6. Johnson YJ, Nickerson M, Quezado ZMN. An unforeseen peril of parental presence during induction of anesthesia. Anesth Anal. 2012;115:1371–2.

Index